Sin or Salvation

Implications for Psychotherapy

Edited by Amy Mahoney and
Oliva M. Espín

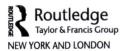

Routledge
Taylor & Francis Group
NEW YORK AND LONDON

First published 2010 in the USA and Canada
by Routledge
270 Madison Avenue, New York, NY 10016

Simultaneously published in the UK
by Routledge
2 Park Square, Milton Park, Abingdon, Oxon, OX14 4RN

Routledge is an imprint of the Taylor & Francis Group, an informa business

© 2010 Taylor & Francis

Typeset in Times by Value Chain, India
Printed and bound in Great Britain by CPI Antony Rowe, Chippenham, Wiltshire

British Library Cataloguing in Publication Data
A catalogue record for this book is available from the British Library

ISBN10: 0-7890-3431-X (hbk)
ISBN10: 0-7890-3432-8 (pbk)

ISBN13: 978-0-7890-3431-1 (hbk)
ISBN13: 978-0-7890-3432-8 (pbk)

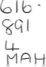

Si

Wh
issu
inte
fills
ther
sexi
pers
cult
pro'
prac
wor

The
wor
are
clin
they

This
wor
lear

This
Fen

Amy Mahoney is a mental health consultant and has worked with homeless, mentally ill women for the past 22 years. She is an active member of several professional organizations including the American Psychological Association (APA), the Association of Women in Psychology (AWP) and the American Association of Service Coordinators (AASC).

Oliva M. Espín is Professor Emerita of Women's Studies at San Diego State University and of Psychology at the California School of Professional Pstchology at Alliant International University.She was a pioneer in the theory and practice of feminist therapy with women from different cultural backgrounds.

CONTENTS

Introduction

Amy Mahoney
Oliva M. Espín

The interplay of women's sexuality and spirituality has seldom been the focus of psychological investigation even though feminist scholars, both psychologists and academic theologians, have written and taught about the necessity of placing women's experience of significant life events at the heart of any investigation of the human experience. There are journals and books that focus on sexuality, and journals and books that focus on spirituality; professional associations concerned with issues of sexuality and those concerned with issues of spirituality. However, sexuality and spirituality are seldom addressed together. The virtual absence of discussions concerning the interplay of sexuality and spirituality in women's lives prompted us to develop this collection. We wanted to invite authors who have worked and reflected on the connections between women's sexuality and spirituality, not just one or the other. The focus of the articles is on how women make meaning of these two, often thought of as separate dimensions of experience.

It is our belief that integration of sexuality and spirituality occurs when previously dichotomized sexuality and spirituality converge. Together, they create a synergistic sexual and spiritual experience that is greater than either separately. Helminiak (1989) argues, "when spirituality is thought to encompass the integration of all aspects of the person and the resultant actualization of one's fullest potential, the role of sexuality in one's spiritual development becomes obvious and pressing" (Helminiak, 1989, p. 201). Indeed, "Carl Jung once remarked that when people brought sexual questions to him they invariably turned out to be religious questions, and when they brought religious questions to him they always turned out to be sexual ones." (Nelson, 1978, p. 14). Jung was not alone in concluding that a person's concerns about sexuality could turn out to be spiritual questions and vice versa.

My (Amy's) interest in exploring the connection between sexuality and spirituality developed precisely because I grew up having been taught there was no connection between the two. I was socialized in the late '40s and '50s in a very strict Irish-American, Catholic, military family in which sex was never discussed but the message was communicated that sexuality meant imitating a virgin mother...an impossible accomplishment! Mixed messages about sexuality and spirituality created for me a chasm impossible to bridge. My parents never talked about sexuality but the Catholic Church preached that sex was only acceptable in marriage and only for procreation. The Catholic Church taught that homosexuality was an abomination to God and a homosexual would never make it into the kingdom of heaven. I was locked out!

My (Oliva's) experience, although very different culturally, is also rooted in Roman Catholic representations of Mary, the mother of Jesus, as the model for "good"–read "submissive and obedient" women, ready to always self-sacrifice for others' sake. But through my personal journey I became aware of other visions and possibilities for women as sexual and spiritual beings. In particular, reading and writing about the women saints of my childhood, has been an eye-opener for me. I have seen how, in the lives of these women, faith and heroism have worked together. I have been captivated by the intricacies of these women's lives, their courage as well as their weakness, their childishness as well as their maturity, their loves and fears, and above all, their focus on doing what they believed God wanted from them regardless of the opinions of others, including the male authorities of Church and family. Their skill in accommodating to and rebelling against patriarchal dictates of the Roman Catholic Church has been illuminating. In a sense their spirituality and mine have grown "against the grain" of traditional beliefs. This understanding has helped me develop a relational spirituality that includes a full acknowledgement of sexuality and connections with fellow human beings. For me, this volume represents another opportunity for learning about the possibilities of integrating sexuality and spirituality.

In Western Christian culture sexuality and spirituality have been dichotomized for hundreds of years. In Psychology, spiritual issues have historically not been seen as the domain of psychological intervention. However, the vast majority of people in the United States have some spiritual belief. An l995 Gallup Poll indicated that 95% of the population of the United States professed some belief in God and approximately 70% professed membership in a church or synagogue. It is, therefore, obvious that spiritual beliefs will be present in the therapy room in one way or another. However, while in most therapeutic approaches the importance of sexuality is not contested, it is isolated from the client's spiritual experiences.

Given the fact that many if not most of our clients will present in therapy with some professed or unexpressed spirituality, the time has come for an integrated approach to the understanding of women's sexuality and spirituality from a feminist psychological perspective. This perspective can facilitate reparative reconnections for women's psycho/sexual/spiritual growth and development. Dualistic, negative thinking that has compartmentalized women's sexuality and spirituality in terms of Madonna or whore needs to be challenged. It is our contention that an integrated, positive understanding of both sexuality and spirituality is needed to empower women to become fully, passionately alive. This is the reason why we decided to collaborate on this topic and invite other feminist therapists to join in. The quality of the articles we have received confirms for us the importance of this topic in feminist therapy.

In this issue, Comas-Díaz discusses the process of uncovering the inner Black Madonna–a feminist psycho-spiritual approach. This process is discussed as an empowering and healing tool. Cultural resonance is explored within what Comas-Díaz calls the intra-ethnic and gender-dyadic therapeutic relationship. Lara describes the work of four Latina health activist-healers whose work challenges the western body/spirit dichotomy from indigenous inspired perspectives. This article is based on Lara's interviews with the four women. She focuses on how these women forward decolonizing feminist perspectives about sexuality and spirituality in their healing/therapeutic work. Stabb et al. present five diverse women therapists who share personal accounts of their own sexuality and spirituality as the starting point for understanding the diverse experiences, both positive and negative, of clients who come to therapy with various degrees of understanding about integration of their sexuality and spirituality. Glassgold discusses the case of an Orthodox Jewish woman who integrated same-sex desire into her life. She describes the psychotherapeutic process in this case and suggests alternative ways of viewing spirituality and sexuality that enable possible resolutions for Orthodox clients. Smith and Horne examine the role of faith, both religion and spirituality, on the sexual satisfaction of lesbian/queer and bisexual women. Mahoney discusses her research exploring the ways in which women socialized in Western Christian culture integrate their sexuality and spirituality. Ogden asks the question: Why do women say no to connecting sex and spirit even when the connection can be self-affirming and potentially life-transforming? She looks for answers in the context of four cultural dynamics (selective education, religious belief systems, norms about pleasure, and mind-body separation) in which women's reluctance to integrate their sexuality and spirituality is rooted. Finally, Daniluk and Browne focus on the differences between religiosity and spirituality, and how women can be assisted to develop more positive and affirming sexual self-constructions and nurture a more empowering sense of spirituality in their lives.

Together, these articles create a picture of what cannot be envisioned yet and what women can achieve in the future in the effort to integrate their sexuality and spirituality. We are proud to present these innovative explorations of women's experiences. We hope this volume will further learning and research on this important topic.

REFERENCES

Helminiak, D.A. (1989). Self-Esteem, Sexual Self-Acceptance, and Spirituality. *Journal of Sex Education & Therapy, 15*(No. 3), 200-210.

Nelson, J.B. (1978). Embodiment: An Approach to Sexuality and Christian Theology. Minneapolis: Augsburg Publishing House.

Our Inner Black Madonna: Reclaiming Sexuality, Embodying Sacredness

Lillian Comas-Díaz

SUMMARY. Feminist therapy needs to acknowledge the role of spirituality in women's lives. The process of uncovering the inner Black Madonna—a feminist psycho-spiritual approach—is discussed as an empowering and healing tool. Clinical material illustrates how the client reclaimed her sexuality and spirituality. Cultural resonance is discussed within the intra ethnic and gender dyadic therapeutic relationship.

For I am the first and the last.
I am the honored one and the scorned one.
I am the whore and the holy one.
I am the wife and the virgin
I am the mother and the daughter....

Lillian Comas-Díaz, PhD, is Clinical Professor at the George Washington University Department of Psychiatry and Behavioral Sciences. She is also in private practice in Washington, DC.

5

I am the barren one,
And many are her sons….
I am the silence that is incomprehensive…
I am the utterance of my name.

–*Thunder, Perfect Mind* (excerpt) Robinson (1990)

INTRODUCTION

Hundreds of icons of the Virgin Mary have black faces. While in France they are called Black Virgins, they are known as Black Madonnas in other countries. The Black Madonna is the iconic remains of the ancient goddess worship syncretized into Christianity. She has been associated with Isis, Black Artemis, Demeter, Cibele (Begg, 1985), Green Tara (Galland, 1990), Kali (Boyer, 2000), and many other dark goddesses. Like her predecessors, she stands for female sexuality in the journey to wholeness (Kidd, 2005). The bearer of the pleasures of love, the Black Madonna is the embodiment of fecundity. Her blackness represents fertility, the color of rich dark soil. When Christianity usurped the goddess, it fragmented and dissociated her qualities, splitting them between the Virgin Mary (immaculate whiteness) and Mary Magdalene, wrongly designated as a whore by early patriarchal church writers (Pagels, 1989). Misogynist clergymen labeled sacred sexuality as prostitution. They suppressed female sexuality and ostracized it from spirituality.

The popularity of the Black Madonna extends to the psychotherapeutic arena (Comas-Díaz, 2003; Mato, 1994; McDermott, 1996). She represents the feminine in man and the self in woman within Jungian psychology (Galland, 1990). As a symbol of inner transformation, the Black Madonna embodies the hidden feminine qualities of healing, intuition, and ancient wisdom. She brings forth, nourishes, protects, heals, receives at death and immortalizes those who follow the way of nature (Begg, 1985). The awakening of the inner Black Madonna facilitates the unfolding of internal guidance.

Contemporary feminists have reinterpreted the Black Madonna as a source of justice, empowerment, reconciliation, and liberation (Castillo, 1996; Comas-Díaz, 2003; Galland, 1990; Mato, 1994; Teish, 1996). The integration of the Black Madonna into our consciousness promotes resilience in the struggle against sexism, oppression, racism, and materialism (Kidd, 2005). In this article, I discuss the psychotherapeutic encounter of a Latina client with a Latina psychotherapist. Utilizing a feminist psycho-spiritual approach, I illustrate the uncovering of the client's inner Black Madonna as a process of recovery and transformation.

DARKNESS ILLUMINATED:
AUREA REACHES THE MOON

Aurea presented to psychotherapy after a breakup with Diego. "I'm not sure I want to be here," she reported. Aurea stated that a female voice in a dream asked her to see a Latina therapist. Upon exploration, the client revealed that she had tried therapy before. "I was ambivalent." A thirty-five-year-old attractive brunette, Aurea was plagued by insomnia and anxiety. "I enjoy men, but can't commit." Upon exploration, Aurea disclosed that she experienced sexual pleasure, but could not achieve orgasm.

Aurea was the older of two daughters. Her parents were Mexicans who met and married after immigrating to the United States. She grew up in a Latino community, where her parents were part of the "servidor" system. Composed of Latinos who use their influential position in the community to benefit others, the "servidor" system functions like an extended family. The owners of a popular bodega, Aurea's parents were in service to others ("servidores") as well as effective community leaders.

Aurea was the first in her family to attend college, and the only one to complete a Ph.D. She secured a tenured academic position as an art historian. The backdrop of her professional success was her history of dramatic losses. At age 12, her parents were in a car accident, where Aurea's mother died while her father was unharmed. "I lost myself that day." Consequently, Aurea assumed the mother's role by taking care of her sister and father. At age 17, she met Rafael and became his girlfriend. Aurea reported that they made love and she achieved orgasm. The romance ended when Rafael drown swimming on Good Friday.

Aurea stopped going to church soon after Rafael's death. "I became an unwed widow." Since he was an only child, Rafael's parents "adopted" Aurea while her father battled alcoholism. At that time, Juan, her older half brother, moved into the family house. Juan became overly involved in raising his half siblings. As a reaction, Nydia, Aurea's younger sister, became a rebellious adolescent, started to abuse alcohol and drugs, and joined a Latino gang.

Aurea became the parental child, the substitute mother, and the caretaker. Her mother's death, her father's emotional abandonment, Juan's intrusiveness, and Nydia's acting out profoundly affected Aurea's ability to sustain attachments. She had several romantic partners, was engaged twice, but broke both engagements. "I am like Dona Flor and her two husbands,' Aurea said, referring to a Brazilian movie with that title. "Rafael's ghost watches over me even if I have a lover." Aurea stated that she could not achieve orgasm with other men. "Only when I am thinking of Rafael," she said.

Aurea's Prophesy

Aurea complained of insomnia and excessive worrying. Her fears seemed connected to bereavement and subsequent loss of control. I used a cognitive behavioral (CBT) approach to help Aurea enhance her sense of agency and mastery. She responded well to the relaxation techniques and systematic desensitization. The therapeutic progress cemented our alliance. Additionally, I suggested mindfulness meditation, an Eastern approach that has been integrated into psychotherapy (Bennett-Goleman, 2001). Indeed, mindfulness has been successfully used in clinical practice for reducing and managing stress (Salmon, Sephton, Weissbecker, Hoover, Ulmer, & Studts, 2004). Moreover, it has been clinically effective in treating abandonment and unlovability schema (Bennett-Goleman, 2001). After challenging her negative schema, we worked on her insomnia. Several trails of behavioral approaches to promote sleep hygiene met with failure. Finally, Aurea stated: "I'm afraid of the dark."

"What do you mean?" I asked.

"When I sleep I see things . . . things that scare me."

"Nightmares?"

"No, I foretell the future in my dreams." Aurea stated that she "saw" Rafael's drowning, her sister's involvement in a gang, and countless events in her dreams before they happened. She felt responsible for the events foretold in her dreams. In particular, Aurea felt that her failure to "protect" Nydia caused her sister to "descend to hell."

I suggested an experiential approach following a mind-body connection to address the prophetic nature of Aurea's dreams. Aurea expressed interest in my suggestion. She revealed that she was a student of Eastern philosophies as well as a yoga practitioner. I introduced the concept of guided imagery or creative visualization stating that it has been used by the ancient Egyptians, Greeks, Native Americans, Chinese Phoenicians, and others long before Carl Jung made it part of depth psychology. I added that guided imagery was commonly used in medicine (Rossman,

2000). I asked her to get familiarized with the topic through the Internet before our next session. Since Aurea was an avid reader, she read several books on the subject before her next appointment. "The ancient Hindu sages believed that images were one of the ways that the gods sent messages to people," she noted.

After helping Aurea get relaxed with progressive muscle relaxation, I introduced the healing light exercise. Borrowed from yoga, this exercise is part of the Eye Movement Desensitization and Reprocessing (EMDR) protocol (Shapiro, 1995). The technique entailed visualizing a vessel (cup, receptacle, vase, etc.) and placing it six inches above the crown of the head. Then, I instructed Aurea to imagine a ray of light the color that she associated with healing. Aurea identified golden yellow as her healing color. The goal was to have the healing light fill her cup, enter Aurea's head, and flow throughout her body. Aurea reported that she felt dizzy during the exercise. I suggested that she ask her healing light to get rid of the dizziness as it traveled throughout her body. Aurea became more relaxed after expressing the request to the healing light. "I'm floating," she said with a smile. After the healing light went throughout her body, I asked Aurea to accompany the light into points in her body that coincide with the seven chakras or energy centers (Brennan, 1988; Fox, 1999; Myss, 1996). Aurea discovered an obstruction in her throat.

"It's a rock in the middle of my throat." Aurea started to hyperventilate.

"Can you shine the healing light into it?" I asked her. "What's happening?"

"The light is breaking the rock. It's pulverizing it."

I continued to guide Aurea through the visualization process.

"My light changed from golden yellow to bright blue," Aurea reported. "The color associated with the throat chakra," she added.

I worked on positive cognitions to counteract Aurea's negative schema. Afterwards, I asked her to repeat the following affirmations:

> I hear and speak the truth.
> I express myself with clear intent.
> Creativity flows through me.
> My voice is necessary.

These affirmations were used to balance her throat chakra. After we completed the guided imagery I recommended specific yoga asanas (postures) for chakra cleansing and balancing. These included the shoulder stand, plough pose, fish pose, head lift and neck rolls (Judith,

1996). Aurea replied that she was going to incorporate these asanas into her yoga routine. We processed the significance of the impediment in her throat during talk psychotherapy. Known as the fifth chakra, the throat energy center is usually associated with communication and with lessons related to will and self-expression (Myss, 1996). I examined Aurea's ability to express her needs within relationships because many women of color adhere to a relational worldview that is central to their sense of healing, well-being, and identity (McGoldrick, García-Preto, Hines, & Lee, 1989). We worked on increasing assertiveness within a Latino cultural context (Comas-Díaz & Duncan, 1985). Aurea used her new assertive style in dealing with her sister Nydia, who notwithstanding her recovery, was still behaving in a dry drunk manner.

"I'm tired of being a substitute mother," Aurea said. She decided to address her co-dependence with Nydia. Moreover, she asked her sister to assume more responsibility.

Sex and the Black Spider

During the next experiential session, I asked Aurea to complete a body scan following the EMDR protocol (Shapiro, 1995). She expressed discomfort in her pubic area. "The light does not flow," she said.

"Can you intensify the light?"

"I see a black spider," she said.

"What's doing there?"

"Prevents me from connecting with pleasure."

We discussed the meaning of the black spider in her pubic area. Aurea disclosed that although her relationships with men had been sexual, she did not experience orgasm. "It was different with Diego," she said. "How?" I asked. "I think I started to fall in love with him," Aurea replied. "But I am an unwed widow," she reminded me, "so I left him."

I asked Aurea to practice asanas (pelvic tilt and cat pose) for balancing her sexual chakra. This chakra is associated with generativity and creativity (Fox, 1999). I explored Aurea's life aspirations during a regular therapy session. "I'm an art critic, but never had the courage to paint," Aurea said. I suggested art classes and encouraged her to follow her bliss. Aurea enrolled in a drawing class and began to bring her creative work into therapy. This suggestion was consistent with the Jungian technique of active imagination, a therapeutic process where the therapist encourages the client to express the images that appear during meditation in an artistic medium (Jacobi, 1948).

"My paintings are missing something," Aurea reported, while showing me her latest work. "What?" I asked. "My heart," she murmured.

I decided to explore Aurea's heart chakra during a guided imagery session. "It's a huge glacier, Aurea said when she saw her heart with her mind's eye. "Just looking at it makes me cold.'

"What do you need?' I asked.

"Melt it with my healing light." Aurea visualized her healing golden yellow light like a beam that melted the glacier sitting on her heart. Interestingly, individuals opening their heart chakra commonly describe the sensation of their chest melting (Fox, 1999). I then asked Aurea to repeat the following affirmations:

> I am worthy of love.
> I am loving to myself and others.
> There is an infinity supply of love.

"I feel lighter," Aurea said after completing the affirmations. "Wait, I see a lake."

"What do you want to do?" I purposely used the word "want" to strengthen Aurea's will.

"Jump into the lake," she replied.

THE DARK WOMAN AT THE BOTTOM OF THE LAKE

Aurea began to swim. "She's calling me," Aurea said.

"Who?" I asked.

"The dark woman at the bottom of the lake."

"Is she your mother?" I remembered Aurea's mother had been morena (dark skinned woman).

"No, she's not Mami, but she's my Mother."

I saw a familiar face of a dark woman with my mind's eye. This revelation reminded me of the Inanna myth, an initiation for women to reconnect with their feminine aspect (Perera, 1981). The myth describes Inanna's (goddess of the heavens) descent into her sister Ereshkigal, the dark goddess queen of the underworld, as a process of death and rebirth. This journey represents feminine renewal and transformation through the integration of the shadow into consciousness. According to Maureen Murdock (1990), women need to reconcile their own repressed mother aspect and integrate it with the masculine before they can achieve a sense of wholeness. Aurea was her mother's age at the moment of her death. My intuition alerted me that the dark face belonged to Aurea's guide. By intuition, I refer to Gary Zukav's (1990) designation of a perception beyond the physical senses that is meant to assist us. I relied on intuition, listening with the third ear to access material that reflects an inner knowing and understanding. Nonetheless, I tried to remain a neutral witness, rationally examining the information before using it. I invited Aurea to make contact with her inner guide. "Not today," she answered.

I did not interpret Aurea's reply. Instead, I took it at face value. According to Deena Metzger (1992), we need to respect the difficulty that some people experience giving up their will to anyone, including to their inner guide. During the following sessions we worked on Aurea's feelings towards her sister. Aurea struggled with guilt and abandonment around Nydia's "descent to hell." Therapy helped Aurea to identify distorted cognitions ("I'm responsible for Nydia's addiction"), distinguish realistic expectations from fantasy ("I will save my sister), and reconcile her ambivalent feelings toward Nydia. She began the transformation of her codependence into self-care and compassionate love.

Aurea brought to therapy an image of a Black woman she sketched. As she discussed her drawing, Aurea recognized the stress of being the same age her mother was at the time of her death. Intuitively, I felt that she was ready to contact her inner advisor. The inner guide (person, animal, object, ancestor, religious/historical figure, etc.) is a form of wisdom and compassion that advises the person. Theologian Thomas Kelly (1941) described contact with the inner guide as the process of uncovering the "eternal internal" by centering down where peace, power, and serenity reside within us. Physicians have used the inner guide technique for healing. For example, in treating cancer, Simonton and his colleagues (1978) taught patients to communicate with their inner guide through visualization or mental imagery for healing advice. Physician Martin Rossman (2000) called this tool the inner advisor. Likewise, psychotherapists have used the inner guide technique. For instance, within CBT, Marsha Linehan (1993) adapted values from Zen, Buddhism, and Taoism, and integrated the "wise mind" into her treatment of people who suffer from borderline personality disorder.

Aurea agreed to contact her inner guide. I followed Metzger (1992) and Rossman's (2000) suggestions for the inner guide meditation. First, I facilitated Aurea's ability to "center" as a way of accessing the synchronicity of mind and body. Then, I guided Aurea into swimming back to the lake.

"Who is your Mother?"

"La Morenita, Guadalupe."

Our Lady of Guadalupe is the patroness of the Americas. Her devotees embrace her as the feminine face of God (Castillo, 1996; Rodriguez, 1996).

"Is she your guide? I asked.

"Yes, she's my Black Madonna," Aurea replied.

"Why is she appearing to you now?"

"Because she has a message" Aurea said. "I'm her child and she loves me. "

"Do you want to ask her something?'

"I did." After a few minutes of silence, tears ran down Aurea's checks.

"What's happening?" I asked Aurea.

"I am sitting on her lap and she's rocking me."

"How are you feeling?"

"Loved." More tears streamed from her eyes.

In *The Secret Gospel of Thomas*, Elaine Pagels (2004) quoted Jesus as saying: "If you bring forth what is within you, what you bring forth will save you. If you do not bring forth what is within you, what you do not bring forth will destroy you" (p. 32). Helping Aurea to bring forth what she had inside was crucial to her healing. Like T. Byram Karasu (2003), I strongly believe that the healer helps by simply helping the client commune with her spiritual nature. However, I was careful not to engage Aurea in an avoidant defense mechanism. Research has found an association between an avoidant attachment to the mother and religious conversion (Kirkpatrick & Shaver, 1990). Indeed, individuals who seek close relationships, but who have difficulty maintaining them due to fears of being unloved and/or abandoned may find the divinity's unconditional love as immensely attractive over romantic relationships (Kirkpatrick, 1999). I strived to help Aurea balance her ability to reclaim herself within relationships. Thus, I recommended the book "Motherless Daughters" (Edelman, 1994) to help her understand the impact of her mother's death on her life.

I addressed Aurea's mourning by helping her connect with her inner Black Madonna. She created several images of Guadalupe. Aurea painted some in Guadalupe's Catholic representation, and others in her indigenous Tonantzin style. I supported this activity because like Tataya Mato (1994), I have found that invoking and drawing the inner Black Madonna is an empowering and healing tool for women. Aurea began to wear a Guadalupe medallion. "This is an offering to my inner Black Madonna," she noted. "It's also a reminder that I'm loved."

THE GOLDEN MORNING MOON

We explored Aurea's prophetic ability during the next therapy phase. Aurea's fears concentrated around her throat chakra. Theologian Matthew Fox (1999) stated that the throat chakra relates to our ability to prophecy because it represents the expression of one's truth and wisdom. Aurea revealed that her mother Selena had a second sight. Aurea experienced prophetic dreams soon after her mother died. The night before her accident, Selena told her daughter why she named her Aurea: "My name Selena means moon and yours means golden. When you were born the first rays of the sun turned the morning moon into gold."

I examined Aurea's negative cognitions regarding her power to prophecy. Aurea revealed that she associated her second sight with "killing" her mother. In other words, not honoring her gift of prophecy helped Aurea to deny her mother's death: "I can't be a motherless daughter and an unwed widow." Aurea connected with her sexual chakra during an experiential session:

"I'm in a temple," she said.

"What's happening?"

"I'm about to have sex."

"How are you feeling?" I asked her.

"I feel nothing."

"Go back into your heart," I suggested. "What do you see?"

"My golden light," Aurea said. "Guadalupe is here."

"Is she communicating with you?"

"She says that she is pregnant with me."

"What's happening?"

"We're dancing." Aurea spontaneously said. "I'm sensual, I'm pleasure, I'm beautiful."

In a memoir about growing up Catholic, Sandra Cisneros (2001) described Guadalupe as a sex goddess. She argued that Tonantzin, her pre-Columbian precursor, embodied all the sex goddesses. For instance, Tlazolteol or Tozin, was the goddess of sex and fertility, as well as the patroness of sexual passion. In her aspect as Tlaelcuani–the filth eater–the goddess could forgive sexual transgressions. Moreover, Cisneros asserted that Guadalupe is Coatlicue, the creative/destructive pre-Columbian goddess. In this aspect Coatlicue-Guadalupe is Kali. Known as a Black one, Kali is the Indian goddess who represents the union of opposites, combining within herself the roles of creation and destruction, birth and death, love and fear (McDermott, 1996).

We worked on Aurea's complicated bereavement during non-experiential sessions. First, we processed Rafael's death. Cognitive behavioral techniques helped Aurea challenge her identity as an unwed widow. She completed the mourning on a Good Friday, the anniversary of Rafael's drowning. Aurea went to church on Easter and felt transformed. She was able to let Rafael go through the Catholic Easter ritual. The timing of the therapeutic work was a coincidence–synchronicity.

We then worked on Aurea's feelings around her father's depression and alcoholism after Selena's death. Aurea was able to forgive her father for driving the car that killed her mother. "I want to reach the morning moon," Aurea announced. "Can you help me?" I facilitated Aurea's visualization of her throat chakra. We used a purification ritual to cleanse her throat from negative cognitions and feelings. Afterwards, Aurea moved into her brow chakra, or third eye, the energy center associated with lessons of the mind, insight, intuition, and wisdom (Brennan, 1988). This chakra is grounded in vision, clairvoyance, and dreams. The challenges of this chakra are to open the mind, develop an impersonal mind, consolidate personal power, learn to act on inner guidance, and discriminate between thoughts motivated by strength and those by fear (Myss, 1996).

"How have you not let yourself be who you are?" I asked Aurea.

"Not loving myself," Aurea said. At that moment, Aurea connected with her inner Black Madonna. She saw Selena placing flowers at Guadalupe's feet.

"What do you want to do?" I asked.

"Sit on my mother's lap." Aurea started to rock. Suddenly, her expression changed.

"What's happening?" I asked.

"La Morenita merged with my mother." Aurea smiled. "They're one." Aurea spontaneously vocalized the following affirmations as she rocked:

> I see all things in clarity.
> I am open to the wisdom within.
> I can manifest my vision.
> I look for the highest and best in all things.

The merging of Guadalupe with Selena appeared consistent with phowa, the Buddhist concept of transference of consciousness. According to China Galland (1990), we can help our mourning by imagining the divinity at the top of the deceased person and sending her positive energy. This spontaneous phowa seemed to open Aurea's third eye (sixth chakra). She became more receptive to guidance and insight through her dreams. I used CBT to reinforce her positive cognitions. Aurea accepted her powers of prophecy. Through mindfulness she began a contemplation practice. As a consequence, Aurea was able to forgive herself for "killing" her mother by accepting her prophetic power. Instead, she was able to identify with Selena. "My mother's spirit is well and alive," she announced. I encouraged Aurea to keep a journal of her dreams.

Aurea reported an increased inspiration in her creative work. Interestingly, Fox (1999) noted that the sixth chakra corresponds to creativity. Indeed, Julia Cameron (2002) identified creative work as a spiritual practice. Aurea brought to therapy a painting depicting a golden morning moon illuminating a girl sitting on her mother's lap.

THERAPIST AS COMADRE

Aurea reported that she started to date Diego, her ex lover. She asked to visualize her pubic chrakra during a guided imagery session: "What do you see?" I asked.

"The spider."

"What do you need to do?"

"Befriend it." Suddenly, Aurea smiled.

"What's happening?" I asked.

"It turned into a star, a bright shining star."

During a regular therapy session, Aurea revealed that she achieved orgasm with Diego. She related her latest dream. "I was giving birth," she said. "You were my comadre." The comadre or co-mother has a central role in the Latino culture. Comadre (co-mother) and compadre (co-father) denote the relationship between the child's godparents and her parents. Compadrazgo is part of allocentrism, a system where members understand themselves through others, emphasize family, social and emotional bonds, and prefer communal goals over individual ones (La Roche, 2002). I interpreted Aurea's dream as a testament of her trust in our therapeutic work. I felt like a comadre in encouraging her transformation.

The intra gender and ethnic therapeutic dyad solidified our working alliance and promoted a cultural holding environment. Such environment helped the emergence of cultural resonance, or the ability to understand clients though a combination of clinical skill, cultural competence, and intuition (Comas-Díaz, 2006). The experiential work further cemented the intuitive aspect of the cultural resonance. Our shared worldview provided psycho-spiritual resonance to therapy. Judith Orloff (1996), a psychiatrist and intuitive, described her clinical intuition–which she called psychic empathy–as the ability to allow the client's feelings to flow through the psychotherapist without over- identifying with them. Joan Koss-Chioino (in press) coined this concept as radical empathy, or the inter-subjective space where intra- and inter-individual differences are melded into one field of feeling and experience in the healing relationship. Conversant in intuitive language, I was able to assist Aurea in her journey to sacred darkness. In my experience, it is important for the psychotherapist to commit to a spiritual practice in order to witness her client's transformation. As an illustration, my inner Black Madonna is a subversive warrior. People struggling for liberation favor the Black Madonna all over the world (Teish, 1996). For me, her darkness represents the inner strength and power of transformation of the oppressed. As a feminist of color, I hear the Black Madonna's call for womanist and mujerista affirmation. Furthermore, the work of Paulo Coelho (2003) on being a spiritual warrior sustained me along this path.

Working with Aurea fortified my vows as a servidora. Aurea's journey was a descent to the goddess–a feminist initiation for women (Perera, 1981). My own heroine's journey (Murdock, 1990) mirrored Aurea's quest for wholeness (Comas-Díaz, 2005a). Working with clients like Aurea reinforced my view of psychotherapy as a profession and a calling (Comas-Díaz, 2005b).

Aurea brought to our last therapy session her sketched version of Frida Khalo's painting depicting the artist giving birth to herself. "I'm my own mother," she announced. Aurea's journey illustrated the integration of feminist therapy with spirituality. Unfolding the inner Black Madonna, a feminist psycho-spiritual approach, promoted recovery, healing, and transformation. It helped Aurea to reconcile the mother-daughter split, reclaim her sexuality, and reconnect with her spirituality.

EPILOGUE: IN THE TIME OF THE BEES

Aurea sent me a package a year after completing therapy. It was a copy of *The Secret Lives of Bees*, a book by Sue Monk Kidd (2002). This best-selling popular novel narrated the story of a motherless daughter who found "home" in the Black Madonna. The book carried a note inside–an invitation. Its cover depicted a golden morning moon illuminating an embracing couple. Aurea was to marry Diego on December 12, the feast of our Lady of Guadalupe. As I turned the invitation to its back, it read: Original work by Aurea Selena.

REFERENCES

Begg, E. (1985). *The cult of the Black Virgin.* London: Arkana/Penguin Books.

Bennett-Goleman, T. (2001). *Emotional alchemy: How the mind can heal the heart.* New York: Harmony Books.

Boyer, M. F. (2000). *The cult of the Virgin: Offerings, ornaments and festivals.* New York: Thames & Hudson.

Brennan, B. A. (1988). *Hands of light: A guide to healing through the human energy field.* New York: Bantam Books.

Cameron, J. (2002). *The artist's way: A spiritual path to higher creativity.* (Tenth anniversary edition). New York: Jeremy P. Tarcher/Putnam.

Castillo, A. (Ed). (1996). *Goddess of the Americas/La Diosa de las Américas: Writings on the Virgin of Guadalupe.* New York: Riverhead Books.

Cisneros, S. (2001). Guadalupe the sex goddess. In M. Sewell (Ed.). *Resurrecting grace: Remembering Catholic childhoods.* (pp. 158-164). Boston: Beacon Press.

Coelho, P. (2003). *Warrior of the Light: A manual.* New York; HarperCollins Publishers.

Comas-Díaz, L. (2003). The Black Madonna: The psychospiritual feminism of Guadalupe, Kali and Monserrat. In L. Silvestein & T.J. Goodrich (Eds.). Feminist Family: Empowerment and social location. (pp. 147-160) Washington, DC. American Psychological Association.

Comas-Díaz, L. (2005 a). In search of the goddess. In V. Ward (Ed). *"Life's Spices From Seasoned Sistahs: A Collection Of Life Spices From Mature Women of Color."* San Francisco: CA. Nubian Images Publishing.

Comas-Díaz, L. (2005 b). Becoming a multicultural psychotherapist: The convergence of culture, ethnicity and gender. *In Session. 61*(2), 973-981.

Comas-Díaz, L. (2006). Cultural variation in the therapeutic relationship. In C. Goodheart R. J. Sternberg &, A. Kazdin, (Eds). *The evidence for psychotherapy: Where practice and research meet.* (pp. 81-105), Washington, DC: American Psychological Association.

Comas-Díaz, L. & Duncan, J. (1985). The cultural context: A factor in assertiveness training with mainland Puerto Rican women. *Psychology of Women Quarterly, 9.* 4. 463-475.

Edelman, H. (1994). *Motherless daughters: The legacy of loss.* New York: A Delta Book, Dell Publishing.

Fox, M. (1999). *Sins of the spirit, blessings of the flesh: Lessons for transforming evil in soul and society.* New York: Three Rivers Press.

Galland, C. (1990). *Longing for darkness: Tara and the Black Madonna.* New York: Compas/Penguin Press.

Karasu, T. B. (2003). *The art of serenity: The path to a joyful life in the best and worst of times.* New York: Simon & Shuster.

Kelly, T. K. (1941). *A testament of devotion.* San Francisco: Harper Collins.

Kidd, S. M. (2002). *The secret life of bees.* New York; Penguin Putnam.

Kidd, S. M. (2005, April 13). *The illuminating Black Madonna.* Lecture presented at the Washington National Cathedral. Washington, DC.

Kirkpatrick, L. A. (1999). Attachment and religious representations and behavior. In J. Cassidy & P. R. Shaver (Eds.), *Handbook of attachment: Theory, research, and clinical applications* (pp. 803-822). New York: Guilford.

Kirkpatrick, L. A., & Shaver, P. R. (1990). Attachment theory and religion: Childhood attachments, religious beliefs, and conversion. *Journal for the Scientific Study of Religion, 29,* 315-334.

Koss-Chioino, J. (in press). Spiritual Transformation and Radical Empathy in ritual healing and therapeutic Relationships, J.D. Koss-Chioino and P. Hefner (Eds.) *Spiritual Transformation and Healing: Anthropological, Theological, Neuroscience and Clinical Perspectives.* Lanham, MD.: Altamira Press.

Jacobi, J. (1948). *The psychology of Jung.* New Haven: Yale University Press.

Judith, A. (1996). *Eastern body, Western mind; Psychology and the Chakra system as a path to the self.* Berkeley, CA: Celestial Arts.

LaRoche, M. J. (2002). Psychotherapeutic considerations in treating Latinos. *Cross-cultural Psychiatry, 10,* 115-122.

Linehan, M. M. (1993). Cognitive-Behavioral Treatment of borderline personality disorder. New York: Guilford Press.

Mato, T. (1994). *The Black Madonna within: Drawings, dreams, reflections.* Chicago: Open Court.

McDermott, R. F. (1996). The Western Kali. In Hawley, J. S. & Wulff, D. M. (Eds.). *Devi: Goddesses of India* (pp. 281-313), Berkeley: University of California Press.

McGoldrick, M.; García-Preto, N.; Hines, P. M.; Lee, E. (1989). Ethnicity and women. In M. McGoldrick; C. M. Anderson; & F. Walsh (Eds.). *Women in families: A framework for family therapy.* New York: Norton.

Metzger, D. (1992). *Writing for your life: A guide and companion to the inner worlds.* San Francisco: Harper Collins.

Murdock, M. (1990). *The heroine's journey: Woman's quest for wholeness.* Boston: Shambhala Publications.

Myss, C. (1996). *Anatomy of the spirit: The seven stages of power and healing.* New York: Three Rivers Press.

Orloff, J. (1996). *Second sight.* New York: Warner Books.

Pagels, E. (1989). *The Gnostic gospels.* New York: Vintage Books.

Pagels, E. (2004). *Beyond belief: The secret gospel of Thomas.* New York: Vintage Books.

Perera, S. B. (1981). *Descent to the goddess: A way of initiation for women.* Toronto: CA: Inner City Books.

Salmon, P., Sephton, S.; Weissbecker, I.; Hoover K.; Ulmer, C.; & Studts, J. (2004). Mindfulness meditation in clinical practice. *Cognitive and Behavioral Practice, 11,* 434-446.

Simonton, O.C. Matthews-Simonton, S. & Creighton, J. (1978). *Getting well again.* New York: Bantam Books.

Shapiro, F. (1995). *Eye movement desensitization and reprocessing: Basic principles, protocols, and procedures.* New York: Guilford.

Robinson, J. M. (1990) (ed), Thunder, perfect mind. *The Nag Hammadi Library*, revised edition. San Francisco: HarperCollins.

Rodriguez, J. (1996). Guadalupe: The feminine face of God. In A. Castillo (Ed.), Goddess *of the Americas/La Diosa de las Américas: Writings on the Virgin of Guadalupe* (pp. 25-31). New York: Riverhead Books.

Rossman, M. L. (2000). *Guided imagery for self-healing: An essential resource for anyone seeking wellness*. Second edition. Tiburon, CA: H.J Kramer.

Teish, L. (1996). The warrior queen: Encounters with a Latin lady. In A. Castillo (Ed.), *Goddess of the Americas/La Diosa de las Americas: Writings on the Virgin of Guadalupe*. (pp. 137-146). New York: Riverhead Books.

Zukav, G. (1990). *The seat of the soul*. New York: Firestone Book (Simon & Schuster).

Latina Health Activist-Healers Bridging Body and Spirit

Irene Lara

SUMMARY. This essay addresses the work of four Latina health activist-healers to show how they challenge the western body/spirit dichotomy from indigenous inspired perspectives that bridge body and spirit, sexuality and spirituality. It discusses some of the ways that Concepción Saucedo, Luz Álvarez Martínez, Angelina Borbón, and Haydeé Rivera Morales forward decolonizing feminist perspectives about sexuality and spirituality through their work as health organization directors, educators, and/or support group leaders. An interview-based analysis, it draws on decolonial feminist methodologies to center these women's voices and interpret their healing work. It concludes with a discussion of the relevance of their health activist-healer work for clinical practice.

Dr. Irene Lara is Assistant Professor of Women's Studies at San Diego State University.

INTRODUCTION

This essay addresses the work of Latina health activist-healers who challenge the western body/spirit dichotomy from indigenous inspired perspectives that bridge body and spirit, sexuality and spirituality. They are working to heal a split that in western cultures can be traced to dominant aspects of medieval Christianity influenced by Greek classical philosophy (Graham, 2001). Indeed, the gendered and racialized binary construction of body/spirit was exacerbated with colonialism as well as the emergence of "scientism" in the 17th century that subordinates the spirit to the body and mind. My research is largely based on qualitative interviews with four women: Concepción (Concha) Saucedo and Luz Álvarez Martínez, based in California's Bay Area, Angelina (Angelita) Borbón, based in Tucson, and Haydeé Rivera Morales, based in New York City. I use "Latina" as an inadequate yet shorthand identity category inclusive of all of the women I interviewed whose racial and ethnic self-referents include Chicana, Mexicana, Puerto Rican, Yaqui, indigenous, and mestiza. Since there is "no all-embracing term acceptable to everyone," I join Elizabeth Martinez who writes, "those of us who seek to build continental unity stubbornly cling to some broadly inclusive way of defining ourselves" (1998, p. 2). I initially interviewed these women in 2001 for an ongoing study on the healing practices and beliefs of twenty-five Latina "healers" (Lara, forthcoming). This essay focuses on the sexual and spiritual aspects of the data collected through these interviews and ongoing communication.

Drawing on and refashioning knowledge from "traditional" indigenous (primarily from the Americas), "modern" western, and hybrid healing beliefs and practices, through their work as health organization directors, advocates, educators, and/or support group leaders, I show how these women embody and forward decolonizing feminist perspectives about sexuality and spirituality. What I mean by decolonizing feminist perspectives is that their work is grounded in a critical historical consciousness that aims to resist and transform the negative impact of racist and sexist ideologies on the lives of women of color. Moreover, I describe these women as activist-healers to highlight that their activism is inseparable from their transgressive healing work and vice-versa. Indeed, their work stems from the desire for personal and social wellbeing. While the range of their activist-healing work is extensive, at the heart of this essay is an analysis of the ways that the activist-healers challenge and transform sexist and eurocentric ideologies by decolonizing the body/spirit split as manifested in Latina's sexuality and spirituality.

In working toward social justice in their communities, Saucedo, Borbón, Rivera Morales, and Álvarez Martínez claim an empowering understanding of spirituality. In doing so, they legitimize an embodied understanding of the spirit and spirituality by recovering and reimagining culturally dynamic indigenous and/or hybrid philosophies that operate from a holistic premise. They view spirituality and sexuality as culturally mediated yet "natural" aspects of being and do not value one over the other or set them in opposition as dominant interpreters of Christianity have done (Jantzen, 2001). In general, the Latinas I interviewed use the term "holistic" to refer to the belief that people's bodies, minds and spirits are connected, that they co-constitute the self, and that when one experiences oneself in this "whole" or connected way, one is more likely to feel that we are all connected. Indeed, this idea is encapsulated by the indigenous philosophy "we are all related to all that lives" (Hernández-Avila, 2002, p. 532). Moreover, as Gloria Anzaldúa (2002) discusses in her notion of "spiritual activism," being holistic impels us to "make the conscious decision to act on our interconnectedness" (Keating, 2005, p. 252). That is, a holistic consciousness behooves these Latinas to act in socially just ways, be it in their everyday lives and relationships, their healing work as counselors and health educators for example, or in more direct social justice organizing work. In addition to equally valuing and integrating the body, mind, and spirit in the consideration of a person's health, for these Latina health activist-healers, working from a holistic health model means taking into account the social and political contexts that impact health.

The healing work of Saucedo, Rivera Morales, Borbón, and Álvarez Martínez is distinct from the work of some activist-healers involved in the politics of women's health because they are grounded in their particular cultural histories that include experiences of racism, classism, homophobia, and sexism. They are part of the tide of "postcolonial" and "multicultural" psychologists, health professionals, public health activists-scholars, and others who forcefully emerged after the Civil Rights movements and addressed the historical neglect of people of color's knowledges, epistemologies, and specific needs in these fields (e.g., Duran & Duran, 1995; Fukuyama & Sevig, 1999). They are rooted in a critical consciousness about the devastating impact colonialism, slavery, imperialism, and patriarchy has wrought on the bodies, minds, and spirits of colonized people and their heirs. For these women of color, colonialism is not abstract or long-ago history. Its legacy is alive, intersecting with sexism, classism, homophobia and other oppressions. It manifests in daily lives through institutional and internalized oppression and dom-

ination and is thus in need of healing. Consciously working from a holistic healing knowledge base that differs from dominant public health
and western biomedical paradigms that focus on the physical nature of
health and disease, yet makes sense to them and their constituents, these
Latinas' activism enacts a "healing logic" (Brady, 2001) that participates
in feminist decolonization.

HELPING LATINA/O COMMUNITIES TO HEAL: CONCEPCIÓN SAUCEDO

Concepción Saucedo is a Chicana-Yaqui psychologist, teacher, community health activist, and *Danza Azteca* (Aztec dance) elder in the San
Francisco Bay Area. The co-founder and recently retired director of the
mental health clinic Instituto Familiar de la Raza servicing the local La-
tino/a community since 1980, she describes her "mission in this life" as
assisting people to discern a "more balanced view of the world and . . .
[our] role as human beings." Many people refer to Saucedo as a spiritual
leader and curandera, a post-colonial healer in the Americas who, in contrast to dominant forms of contemporary Western medicine, treats the
body, mind, and spirit in relationship to each other (Avila, 1999). However, she humbly acknowledges "whatever gifts [she's] been given . . . to
be a teacher and to help people heal" and chooses not to call herself any of
those honorific titles. Yaqui and Mexica (Aztec) oral knowledges, as well
as her graduate study of Northern American and Mesoamerican history
and anthropology, influence Saucedo's ideas about healing, spirituality,
and sexuality. Saucedo's values were impacted by her parents "who still
carried some of their own native traditional practices" and were involved in
social justice work. In the early, 1970s Saucedo began meeting with like-
minded colleagues to collectively "try to relearn" indigenous knowledges.
This was the seed that grew into the founding of Instituto Familiar de la
Raza. In addition to her status as a community intellectual grounded in
indigenous knowledges, Saucedo has a Doctorate in Psychology.

Defining spirituality as "any experience that connects us to . . . that
which is larger than us . . . the Creator, that divinity or that universality . . .
whatever this unknown is of energy," at the center of Saucedo's everyday life and healing work are her spiritual worldviews. For example,
Saucedo works toward embodying the Mayan concept of *In Lak'ech* (I
am your other I). This worldview, she explains, "says we are all related
to everybody and every creature and every aspect of the environment."
She integrates her psychology training, indigenous philosophies about

the social and cosmic role of the human, and *curanderismo* healing practices such as *limpias* (sprit cleansings) and ceremony, with her clients and interns at Instituto Familiar (e.g., Avila, 1999). Viewing dominant psychology models as limiting, she also (re)trains psychologists, nurses, and social workers using a pedagogical model inspired by the pre-colonial Mexica center of education that taught spiritual and healing knowledge, the "*calmécac*" (León-Portilla, 1963).

In addition to her psychology healing work, Saucedo is an educator in all of her roles, including as a public speaker, teacher and spiritual leader for local *danza* groups, and ex-college professor. Integral aspects of the indigenous spiritual knowledges that Saucedo teaches in her various capacities are her decolonizing ideas about sexuality and the body. Although some historians believe that abortion "was at least in theory harshly punished" (Wiesner-Hanks, 2000, p. 145), Saucedo draws from her oral traditions to provide a view of abortion as a woman's own decision: "In Native cultures, abortion always existed. There were *yerbas* [herbs] that we used to abort if that was necessary. It doesn't look like it's a sin against anybody, because sin didn't exist in that way. We had knowledge that some spirits come into the world, but then [sometimes] it's not their time, so they're not to be born." She elaborates her decolonial perspective, "And . . . yes, [sex] can be pleasurable. I think the Catholic Church kind of messed us up on that one; [by teaching] that it's not supposed to be pleasurable and it was [only] supposed to be at certain times." Indeed, in contrast to such indigenous views, Christian teachings have historically been interpreted as subordinating the body and earthly concerns (conceptually linked with females) to the spirit and spiritual concerns (conceptually linked with males) (Jantzen, 2001). Invoking the oral teachings of Mexica wise old men and women, Saucedo emphasizes that they taught both females and males, "You're on this earth, and you will have pain and suffering, but Creator leaves you the beauty of sexuality and it leaves you song. It leaves you beauty to make your time here on Earth pass better." Such extant beliefs are also documented in colonial texts further suggesting the popularity of what is arguably an empowering view of female sexual pleasure (Marcos, 1991). However, Mexica female sexuality was often, though not exclusively, couched within a heteronormative reproduction framework (Clendinnen, 1991; López Austin, 1980). Regardless, Saucedo's contemporary reinscription expands beyond this focus.

In spite of this Native legacy, because of the views imposed by Catholic colonialism, claims Saucedo, "[W]e've forgotten [this view of sex] that got overlaid with…Catholic teachings that come from . . . [a] patriarchal view." Although patriarchy is arguably part of many indigenous cultures, particularly imperialistic ones, Saucedo thinks that "still among more traditional, more Native people, [sex] is just a natural thing and you should not be ashamed or embarrassed by it or by those yearnings that we have." For many, but certainly not all, Native American, Mesoamerican, as well as African indigenous cultures, this affirming view of sexuality has included valuing what western culture has termed homosexuality and gender crossing. Although homophobia is currently part of many indigenous communities, such "two-spirit people," Saucedo teaches, were once highly esteemed by their communities for having "spiritual insights into the spirit world that other people didn't [or don't] have" (see, e.g., Fukiyama & Sevig, 1999, p. 127).

Catholicism's virgin/whore dichotomy has been particularly pervasive as a control mechanism and thus detrimental to the expression of female sexual desire and pleasure in general, and non-married and queer sex in particular. As Saucedo explains, when women are "given a 'Virgin' [to emulate] that is a virgin, then you begin setting up [the ultimatum] 'if you don't behave like this Virgin, you are *la Puta* [the Whore].'" Within a colonial context, white women were more likely to have access to virginity and thus its attendant social status while indigenous and other women of color–who were more likely to be raped and in illicit, unmarried relationships–were less likely to embody this privilege. Race and class, therefore, also differentiate this dichotomy (Espín, 1997a). This culturally constructed dichotomy divides "good" from "bad" Latina women along the lines of their sexual behavior, leaving little room for "good" alternatives beyond virginity and marriage. Lamenting on the impact of dominant Catholic colonial thought, Saucedo elaborates, "So if you dare, say, enjoy [sex], then you have to be a *puta*, right? And those were so contrary to the views, I think, of Native people."

Through her various health activist-healer roles, Saucedo encourages awareness about some empowering indigenous conceptions of the sexual female body-spirit. By learning how our dominant gendered, classed and racialized worldviews about sexuality are part of a generally oppressive Catholic colonial legacy, psychologists and others in healing roles can be better informed about how their own ideas about sexuality as distinct from one's spirituality are culturally constructed. By enabling them to recognize and understand their clients when they speak from indigenous and/or Catholic worldviews, this knowledge will help healers address their clients' needs. Moreover, they can share this knowledge with women whom they are trying to help heal from, for example, internalized shame for "bad" sexual behavior.

AWAKENING CONSCIOUSNESS
VIA LA COMADRE CONCIENCIA:
ANGELITA BORBÓN

Angelita Borbón, who identifies as a mestiza-Yaqui Indian from the Sonoran desert, has been a nurse and health educator for more than twenty years and is contemplating enrolling in a doctoral nursing program. Borbón participated in the, 1970s wave of women's health activism after learning about the death of a woman who had an illegal abortion. Enraged into action, Borbón began helping women have access to legal abortions and teaching women about sex, sexual anatomy, and the reproductive system. Although she considers herself a "conceptualizer" of health and indigenous and mestiza healing and not an activist or "healer per se," I interpret such conceptualizing work as a significant aspect of health activist-healing work. Resonating with the cultural grounding of Saucedo's activism, Borbón draws from her mestiza-Yaqui family heritage and the indigenous oral traditions of Teotihuacan that she began studying in Mexico in 1978.

Elaborating her spiritual worldview, Borbón says, "I think my role is to…awaken consciousness and to help people remember how to be in the world, [remember] their relationship with the cosmos, remember how it is they want to be, and help them to feel and understand their relationship to everything else, the fact that all things are connected, that we are the web that connects us." Integral to this process of "*despertando conciencia*" (awakening consciousness) is shedding the multiple "masks," including colonial masks, that get in the way of this holistic knowing. Lest we misinterpret her work as a naïve call for mestizas/os and indigenous people to return to life before colonialism, Borbón's focus is on practicing what she terms a "*comadre consciencia*" as an authentic yet dynamic way of being that will help "people survive" in contemporary contexts. Borbón describes being in the role of "*comadre*," which she defines as a chosen sister, in her many "jobs" throughout the last 25 years or so. Literally Spanish for "co-mother," *comadre* denotes chosen kinship within a spiritual framework. As Borbón conceptualizes it, a *comadre* is a support person during the birthing, nurturing, and survival process, be it of a person or a creative expression. For Borbón, this includes being a doula, "a woman who assists another woman during labor and provides support to her, the infant, and the family after childbirth" (*Webster's*), reproductive justice activist, nurse, teacher to nurses, medical residents, physicians, and pregnant women, public speaker, daughter, mother, grandmother, and other "things [she's] chosen to put [her] energy into" in her daily life.

Teaching from a perspective that considers the reproductive aspects of sexuality, including pregnancy and childbirth, Borbón forwards a decolonizing view about spirituality and sexuality that heals the western split between body (or "heart") and mind. She recounts her experience with teaching "Preparing for Birth" to Spanish-speaking immigrants:

> Many of the immigrants are in their bodies; their experience of life is in their bodies . . . And then they go to a [western] traditional preparation for childbirth class and they start teaching them how to do breathing patterns and counting…and they put them in their heads . . . So the classes I've been able to teach are about just listening to your body in birth, getting into the natural rhythms that your body will get you into, and relating those to things like waves in the ocean and other powerful, natural phenomena. [My classes are about] keeping them in their bodies, as opposed to disassociating them, because that's what this culture teaches–a break between the head and the heart–and that's not our natural way.

By claiming her indigenous, mestiza "cultural, historical heritage [which] is to be of heart and mind," Borbón counters the "break" that has become common in post-Enlightenment thought and suggests that a holistic approach can be more empowering to birthing mothers.

As a "*comadre*" in all aspects of her life, Borbón's conceptual framework is built on "indigenous values opposed to colonial values." For Borbón, this means that sexuality and spirituality are related because they are both integral aspects of the self. Borbón believes,

> [S]exuality is just one component of how we relate in the world. It's just a very real part of our expression and unfortunately [in western culture] it's become a commodity, something you use to negotiate . . . instead of just an expression like laughter and dancing and a hug and conversation . . . It's taken on "dark" [and] "the other" perspectives, and so sexuality functions in the dark in a lot of ways instead of being just an open part of our expression.

Moreover, Borbón does not separate all of the "vaginal politics" work she has participated in from her spirituality. When I asked, "How do you integrate your indigenous Mexican philosophies with your 'vaginal politics' work?" Borbón responded, "I have no way of separating out anything from my 'spirituality,' not even vaginal politics. I think maybe the question itself is looking for a connection when there are not separate entities to 'connect'" (personal communication, 16 February, 2003).

Borbón's conceptualization of one's sexuality and body as inseparable from one's spirituality and spirit can be helpful to better understand the splitting, violent impact of sexual abuse and, therefore, help heal such wounds. As Borbón states, "So if your body has been treated like a sexual object . . . or if you're like so many women who've been abused and violated violently . . . I think it would be easy to disassociate from [your] body because [your] body would carry those painful memories. In which case then, where's the spirit in that? And I think that is something that really needs to be healed." Although Borbón's *comadre conciencia* work has not directly dealt with healing sexual violence, her views may be conceptually helpful in understanding and healing the effects of such violence. As bodies and spirits, women's experiences of sexual violence may impact their spiritual wellbeing in addition to their physical and mental wellbeing. As also addressed by curandera and nurse Elena Avila (1999), this holistic perspective can help some survivors of sexual violence heal. Moreover, it can help loved ones and counselors better support survivors.

PROMOTING COMMUNITY HEALING AND SELF-HEALING: HAYDEÉ RIVERA MORALES

Haydeé Rivera Morales describes herself as a Puerto Rican mother of working class background born and raised in New York City. In 1994, she co-founded Casa Atabex Aché, a health organization for women of color in New York City that promotes "self-healing" work in connection to social justice, and was its director from 1999 to 2002. Resolute about the difference between Casa's self-healing model and self-help models that do not connect the self to social change and perpetuate "individualism as opposed to collectivism healing," at "the heart of" Casa's work, says Rivera Morales, is "changing the world through an individual journey which impacts the family which will impact the community." Through "Healing Circles" (support groups), peer counseling, and health education workshops such as "The Erotic Health Party," the aim of self-healing is to "[free] oneself from one's own internalized oppression... [and] self-hate." A decolonizing and feminist political approach threads through all of Casa's programs which aim to provide "the opportunities and resources for womyn to reclaim their bodies, minds and spirits and as a consequence their rights" (http://www. casaatabexache.org/index.php?name=whycasa).

Dismayed by the health education models she learned as a Community Health major and Human Services Administration master's student that did not adequately address the social realities of people of color, Rivera Morales attributes much of her consciousness to her experiences with the First World Women of Color Healing Circle. Emerging from people of color health movements, this group of New York City women of color healers–including midwives, massage therapists, teachers, Chinese medicine doctors, acupuncturists, Reiki practitioners, and community organizers–came together from the end of the 1980s to 1995 to do "seasonal fasting and emotional healing so that they could go back to their communities and continue the [healing] work." Serving as a genesis to Casa Atabex Aché, this Healing Circle taught Rivera Morales how self-healing and social change are linked as well as the importance of emotionally healing work. She discusses her own healing experience as an example of its transformative power:

> I'm a survivor of childhood sexual abuse. . . . [A]s I grew up, because I had not dealt with that pain, I had very painful periods. I would throw up. I would get diarrhea. I would pass out and just be in excruciating pain for seven days . . . I went to the doctors and they put me on the pill and they put me on Depo-Provera . . . they told me I couldn't have kids . . . It wasn't until I came to the First World Woman of Color Healing Circle and . . . dealt with the pain . . . and the rage of being victimized for so many years, then all of a sudden I had periods that were painless . . . And I have [my daughter] Marcela now.

Rivera Morales's own self-healing work coincided with establishing Casa Atabex Aché, where she helped to facilitate the self-healing work of hundreds of women every year.

The self-healing model is grounded in the thesis that, states Rivera Morales, "[W]e're born into this world perfect but what happens is as soon as we come into this world we are introduced to elements of oppression," such as the imposition of gender roles, other forms of sexism, heterosexism, racism, and classism. The peer-education counseling model provides a collective space for people to express their experiences of oppression by telling their stories, crying, yelling, or other forms of emoting. Working in groups of a minimum of three people, one person releases and another supportively listens and encourages the release, while a third person supports both the women while sitting or standing behind or next to them. In contrast to uni-directional individual counseling, such as in the dominant psychotherapy model where there is a therapist treating a client, Casa uses a model in which everyone takes a turn emoting their feelings. Morales Rivera elaborates on the reasons for this approach: "[W]e feel it's much more powerful that a woman heals, let's say from sexual abuse, in collective space. Because then it gives permission for other women to break the silence as well, than if we just do it with one person." Moreover, akin to other group counseling models popularized with the advent of consciousness raising groups and the feminist understanding that "the personal is political," this method shows women that "this is not happening to me, it's happening to us." This social consciousness can inspire women to participate in social change.

In describing Casa's self-healing model, Rivera Morales redefines what is dominantly constructed as spirituality by focusing on what she calls internal sources of power, women's "essence" or "life-source." Challenging patriarchal definitions of spirituality that rely on external and male sources of power, as well as "woman-centered Goddess-y" models that do not consider the "connection to one's internal life force," Rivera Morales and Casa are teaching women, "[Y]ou already have the strength, you already have the power, it's innate, you were born with it and it's about tapping in[to] . . . and operating from that place." This model is "combating internalized oppression," says Rivera Morales, by "really helping women to understand the power that they have internally and connecting to that light . . . fire . . . vibration . . . energy . . . whatever you want to call it" rather than only looking outside themselves for spiritual power. Part of the decolonization of spirituality and sexuality away from their patriarchal and racist hold is Casa's engagement with Caribbean and African indigenous "fertility Goddesses," Atabex and Akua. By engaging female-centered, earth-based beliefs they are transforming some of the largely Christian-based community members' racist judgments that often demonize "anything . . . associated to the African diaspora." Reflecting on her own experiences and the self-healing work that she has facilitated, Rivera Morales believes, "whatever connection one has to a 'spiritual' source that is not oppressive will create some level of healthy self-love that will then manifest in healthy sexuality."

While the self-healing model generally addresses spirituality and sexuality from a decolonizing feminist perspective, one of Casa's many programs that directly addresses these issues is "The Erotic Health Party" held for many years in a woodsy retreat center where women's self-healing is believed to be facilitated by being in an earthy, "spiritual" environment. Integrating health education and healing work, the erotic is presented in relation to issues of power, both in terms of the ways women experience sexual violence and dominance and the ways the erotic, as profoundly articulated by Audre Lorde (1984), is an internal source of power to be acknowledged and reclaimed. As Rivera Morales describes,

> [W]e are promoting safer sex but also making it very erotic so that it's not just, "This is how you put a condom on a penis" and "This is how you use a dental dam" . . . [W]e're introducing whipped cream and strawberries and feathers . . . [W]e're [also] talking actively about the violence in our lives . . . and really using the exercise of health promotion through the erotic as a reclaiming of those parts of oneself that may have been abused either by self through internalized oppression or through our oppressive world.

Raising consciousness about the ways that women's erotic power has "historically been targeted for violence and for domination and control," such as through rape, sexual abuse, sexual harassment, and battering, is part of resisting and healing sexual oppression.

In providing opportunities for consciousness raising and self-healing work that holistically focuses on Latinas' lives, Casa Atabex Aché is challenging racialized and sexualized representations of Latinas as perpetuated by mainstream culture and oftentimes internalized by Latinas themselves. Raising consciousness about the role of (neo)colonialism, racism, classism, and sexism in the construction of such monolithic portrayals, as well as self-healing work that heals internalized oppressions, helps women connect to their agency. By promoting a holistic attitude toward spirit, sex, self-pleasure, pleasuring men and/or women, and providing spaces where women can heal, from sexual abuse or other issues, Rivera Morales and the rest of Casa Atabex Aché's staff works to bridge the body and the spirit and decolonize the sex/spirit split.

PROMOTING HOLISTIC HEALTH EDUCATION: LUZ ÁLVAREZ MARTÍNEZ

Luz Álvarez Martínez, co-founder and director of the Oakland, California-based National Latina Health Organization (NLHO) since its founding in 1986 until 2005, describes her role as a holistic health advocate and educator as spiritual and political healing work. She identifies as an *indígena* (indigenous woman), Chicana, Latina, *danzante*, spiritual person, and activist. Raised Catholic, Álvarez Martínez left the Church soon after starting a family and confronting the tension between experiencing sex as natural, pleasurable, and in her control and institutional dogma that questioned her guilt-free sexuality and demanded that she reject birth control. A primary source of her indigenous worldview about "the interconnectedness of everything" and maintaining her own holistic wellbeing comes from participating in the *Danza Azteca* community since 1991. It was then that Álvarez Martínez began understanding her health activist-healer work as part of her spirituality, which she defines as "everything about you, the way you do your life." A key aspect of Álvarez Martínez' leadership in the NLHO is "promoting Self-Help as a tool for individual empowerment and social change" (Gutierrez, 2004, p. 243) through a holistic approach to Latina health. Although Álvarez Martínez is involved in a wide array of health activism that bridges body and spirit, I focus my discussion on the NLHO's Intergenerational Latina Health Leadership Project, "a revolutionary model for holistic health education" that crosses the modern borders between communities inside and outside of the university (Ayala, Herrera, Jiménez, & Lara, 2006).

The Intergenerational Latina Health Leadership Project was comprised of college courses and conferences. "Redefining Latina Health: Body, Mind, Spirit," taught at the University of California, Berkeley (in 1998, 1999, and 2004) and Hunter College-City University of New York (from 2000 to 2003), was co-created by Álvarez Martínez, NLHO staff, and graduate students (including myself), with input from undergraduates. The course content, that includes topics such as "Spiritualities," "Sexuality and Power," and "Reproductive Justice," was consciously organized to foreground women-centered, decolonizing perspectives about Latina lives and health.

In addition to addressing sterilization abuse, the harmful effects of contraception methods such as Depo-Provera, and other Latina reproductive justice issues, Álvarez Martínez's public presentations dispelled the social myth that all or most Latinas are adamantly opposed to contraception and abortion. Moreover, she worked toward healing the shame often internalized by women who use contraception or have had abortions. She recalls hesitating to tell her mother, a devout Catholic immigrant from Mexico, about her increasingly public involvement with the National Abortion Rights Action League and other pro-choice activism.

To Álvarez Martínez' surprise, her mother approvingly responded with, "*¿Pues si la mujer no tiene eso, qué tiene?* [Well, if a woman doesn't have that (the right to terminate her own pregnancy), what does she have?]." As also discussed by Saucedo, abortion has been widely practiced by women in the Americas before and after colonialism, in spite of the Catholic orthodoxy's admonitions. In fact, as Álvarez Martínez also discusses in her lectures, the Church did not construct abortion as sinful until after the mid-nineteenth century (Wiesner-Hanks, 2000). Indeed, although there is strong evidence showing a pattern of support for abortion rights by Latinas, the dominance of a Christian worldview has arguably contributed to public silence about abortion (Pesquera & Segura, 1998).

As with all NLHO programs, Álvarez Martínez was instrumental in incorporating Self-Help, the NLHO's peer-counseling process that facilitates "individual empowerment and social change" (Gutierrez, 2004, p. 243), into the class, as well as the conferences. As analyzed in Ayala, Herrera, Jiménez, & Lara (2006), pedagogically using this process (akin to Casa's self-healing model) created opportunities for students to feel more comfortable expressing their own experiences with abortion, and sex and sexuality in general. Indeed, her talk the two years I was a co-instructor launched a series of passionate class discussions, writings by students, and self-disclosures. As described in an article co-written by four of the class instructors, the opportunity to publicly articulate personal experiences was "a step for [students] in healing the shame that's perpetuated about abortion" (Ayala, Herrera, Jiménez, & Lara, 2006, p. 276).

The two conferences, "*Haciendosé Mujeres* [Becoming Women]: A Celebration of Latinas Coming of Age" held in 1999 and 2000, were also collectively structured to present a holistic view of health that intergenerationally engaged Latinas' spiritualities and sexualities. Conference workshops included: Desire and the Erotic: Beyond "Sex"; Lesbian Sexual Health; What Is a Pelvic Exam? Visiting the Gynecologist; If You Could See Her in the Mirror, What Would She Look Like? Pussyology; STD's and HIV/AIDS; and Traditional and Nutritional Approaches to Health and Reproductive Health. The conferences were organized with a special focus on the physical maturation of Latina adolescents in ways that celebrate female sexuality and challenge the sexual silences often sanctified by family, school, and the Church (Zavella, 2002). For example, Saucedo, a keynote presenter at the first conference, conducted a ceremony based on indigenous Mexican traditions, including burning *copal* (incense) and praying to the four directions, and discussed an indigenous worldview that values women's life cycle from birth to death. During her talk she emphasized the importance of maintaining balance in one's life, that taking care of one's spiritual and mental health is just as important as taking care of one's physical health, and that imbalance in one affects the whole. Another challenge to the social silences and distortions about Latina women's sexuality, Álvarez Martínez describes Saucedo's indigenous-inspired presentation of sexuality as "a natural part of who we are. It's nothing to be ashamed of. It's nothing to be secretive about. It is a natural, beautiful part of our lives."

This perspective also accurately describes another speaker's message at the first conference. Dr. Cindy Grijalva, an Ecuadorian-American obstetrician-gynecologist, gave a western medical perspective on women's reproductive anatomy and health yet discussed the importance of valuing Latina's culturally different ways of understanding women's bodies. She stirred the morning audience of about 150 people with an actual speculum, slides of women's genitalia and reproductive system, and a Mexica image of a woman giving birth. As Grijalva explained, the Mexica gave first-time birthing women the status of valiant warriors; in the case of their death, they would go directly to heaven. Also integrated by Borbón into her presentations, such a worldview that links sexuality and spirituality can be interpreted as empowering birthing mothers with respect for their life and death work. Lest we overly romanticize the "idea that women giving birth were fighting death"–which is still very much the reality where there is a high incidence of maternal and infant mortality–however, it is important to think about how this idea may have also perpetuated the expectation that women had to be martyr-like mothers. Borbón adds that indigenous midwives were also considered warriors for "assisting women in . . . their valiant effort." She explains, "[W]hen the baby was born, the midwife gave a cry . . . the same cry that was given when a warrior was victorious on the battlefield . . . that let everyone know that the woman had vanquished death and had brought forth life."

Beyond only addressing reproduction and birthing, however, both Grijalva and Saucedo beautifully communicated some of the messages Álvarez Martínez hoped the conference would convey: that sexuality, be it heterosexuality, homosexuality, or other sexualities on the continuum, is a natural, indeed spiritual, part of the human experience; and that sex should be pleasurable for all involved. The conference keynotes, as well as the eighteen workshops participants had to choose from, provided an alternative to some Christian beliefs that primarily link sex to heterosexual reproduction within marriage and view the sexual (especially female and/or queer) body as essentially contaminated

(Jantzen, 2001). Moreover, it went beyond an uncritical "exaltation of the virtue of reproduction" (López Austin, 1988, p. 303) found in Spanish colonial documents about the Mexica and other indigenous groups by also celebrating sexuality beyond procreation. Finally, this health activism-healing work serves as an example of socially addressing Latina sexualities and spiritualities in decolonizing feminist ways.

Many lives have been touched by Álvarez Martínez's commitment to empowering Latinas intergenerationally and by bridging communities inside and outside of the university. As one of the graduate students who worked with the NLHO's Intergenerational Latina Health Project, participated in Self-Help trainings, and co-taught "Redefining Latina Health: Body, Mind, and Spirit," I can testify to the personally healing impact of NLHO's work under Álvarez Martinez's leadership. In fact, my commitment to forwarding decolonizing feminist views on spirituality and sexuality and personal and social wellness has been inspired and supported through my experiences with the NLHO and Álvarez Martinez's mentorship.

CONCLUSIONS AND RELEVANCE FOR CLINICAL PRACTICE

These Latina health activist-healers are addressing spirituality and sexuality in feminist and decolonizing ways that are empowering to themselves and others in their communities. They challenge patriarchal and eurocentric hegemony on various levels. For example, by bringing a feminist perspective to the work they do, they raise consciousness about the structures of sexism and how internalized sexism works. As importantly, they provide opportunities for emotionally discharging and reflecting on how patriarchy has impacted Latinas' lives and thus for healing and transforming patriarchy's effects (e.g., Espín, 1997b; Rodriguez, 2001). By bringing a decolonial perspective to the work they do, they are also raising consciousness about the historical legacies of colonialism, Christianity, and eurocentrism in constructing their beliefs and practices. This perspective provides their constituents with the opportunity to then rethink and better understand their beliefs and practices, while teaching them the healing aspects of their historically demeaned indigenous and African cultures. Like other healers and activists who empower women, their liberatory work poses a threat to the status-quo—be it patriarchy, Christianity, eurocentrism, heterosexism, or any combination thereof—and hence they face criticism and resistance. Yet, guided by their vision for holistic wellness in their communities and the broader global community, and strengthened by their own commitment to continually work on healing themselves, they persist with their activist-healer work.

It is my contention that western oriented therapists may benefit from reflecting on these Latina's cultural perspectives and practices as examples of holistic approaches to addressing healing and wellbeing within a social context. Saucedo suggests that being truly culturally competent when working with Latino/as requires more than learning about their holistic beliefs and practices from a textbook; it is essential to respectfully engage and integrate such perspectives into one's work. As educators for example, these Latinas do not only teach these worldviews that bridge body, mind and spirit and decolonize sexuality and spirituality, they also aim to teach this in an integrated way, from bodymindspirit. Indeed, Saucedo, Borbón, Rivera Morales, and Álvarez Martínez aim to model in their lives what they are teaching. Therapists interested in learning such worldviews should respectfully seek teachers, beginning with contacting local Latina/o health organizations. Therapists who are affiliated with universities can also participate in structural change by recruiting, hiring, and supporting teachers and students with such knowledges.

Moreover, emphasizing that cultural competency must include learning about privilege, Álvarez Martínez questions the value of learning "our culture" without unlearning racism, classism, and other oppressions. Indeed, the four Latina health activist-healers in my study join others in emphasizing the need for therapists to have "an analysis of the social world...[that] includes an understanding of the impact of oppression due to gender, race, ethnicity, class, sexual orientation, disability, and age" (Espín, 1997b, p.68). As Oliva Espín asserts, a good therapist also needs to understand "the impact of privilege on the lives of those who do not belong to oppressed groups in these categories" (p. 68). Given that consciousness is a continual process, these Latinas also accentuate that therapists themselves need to consistently work on the ways they have internalized oppression and privilege so that they do not perpetuate them. As Saucedo articulates, by virtue of being recognized as "healers," people in counseling roles have power and need to be self-vigilant about not abusing that power. Indeed, these Latinas believe that healers are in need of healing. When I asked two of the interviewees what they would want therapists to learn from their work, they both highlighted the need for all healers to "do their work" to heal internalized dominance and oppression. Having experienced oppression from western oriented therapists and teachers, they stressed that it is not enough for therapists to participate in a few cultural competency or anti-racism trainings. As Rivera Morales states, healing from internalized privilege, like healing from internalized oppression, is a continual process because although "we change" as we work on healing ourselves and unlearning privilege and oppression, "the world around you hasn't."

Future research would benefit from interviewing more Latinas involved in similar healing work throughout the U.S. Moreover, it would be helpful to interview the beneficiaries of such work in order to determine the work's efficacy beyond the self-reports of the women I interviewed. In order to have a better understanding of the ways that the body and spirit, sexuality and spirituality are split and integrated by Latinas of all sexual orientations, prospective studies should also include interviews with health-activists who are more directly addressing lesbian, bisexual, and transgender sexuality in their work.

END NOTE

I have much gratitude for Concha, Angelita, Haydeé, and Luz, the four women whose theories and practices are the heart of this study. I also give thanks to Oliva Espín, Laura Jiménez, and Sophia Arredondo for feedback during various stages of this paper and Jessica Far for help with references. Mil gracias to my family, especially Raúl Trejo, Dolores Lara, and Edda Trejo, the loving caretakers of my daughter Belén who help make my scholarly work possible and pleasurable.

REFERENCES

Anzaldúa, G. (2002). Now let us shift....the path of conocimiento....inner work, public acts. In G. Anzaldúa & A. Keating (Eds.), *this bridge we call home: radical visions of transformation* (pp. 540-578). New York: Routledge Press.

Avila, E. (with Parker, J.). (1999). *Woman who glows in the dark: A curandera reveals traditional Aztec secrets of physical and spiritual health*. New York: Tarcher/Putnam.

Ayala, J., Jiménez, L., Herrera, P., & Lara, I. (2006). Fiera, guambra, y karichina! Transgressing the borders of community and academy. In D. Delgado Bernal, C. A. Elenes, F. E. Godinez, & S. Villenas (Eds.), *Chicana/Latina education in everyday life: Feminista perspectives on pedagogy and epistemology* (pp.261-280). Albany: State University of New York.

Brady, E. (Ed.). (2001). *Healing logics: Culture and medicine in modern health belief systems*. Logan: Utah State University Press.

Clendinnen, I. (1991). *Aztecs: An interpretation*. Cambridge: Cambridge University Press.

Duran, E., & Duran, B. (1995). *Native American postcolonial psychology*. Albany: State University of New York Press.

Espín, O. M. (1997a). Cultural and historical influences on sexuality in Hispanic/Latin women: Implications for psychotherapy. In *Latina realities: Essays on healing, migration, and sexuality* (pp. 83-96). Boulder: Westview Press.

Espín, O. M. (1997b). Feminist approaches to therapy with women of color. In *Latina realities: Essays on healing, migration, and sexuality* (pp. 51-70). Boulder: Westview Press.

Fukuyama, M. A. & Sevig, T.D. (1999). *Integrating spirituality into multicultural counseling*. Thousand Oaks: Sage Press.

Graham, H. (2001). *Soul medicine: Restoring the spirit to healing*. Dublin: Newleaf.

Gutierrez, E. (2004). National Latina health organization. In J. Silliman, M.G. Fried, L. Ross, & E. Gutierrez (Eds.), *Undivided rights: Women of color organize for reproductive justice* (pp. 241-261). Boston: South End Press.

Hernández-Ávila, I. (2002). In the presence of spirit(s): A meditation on the politics of solidarity and transformation. In G. Anzaldúa & A. Keating (Eds.), *This bridge we call home: radical visions of transformation* (pp. 530-538). New York: Routledge Press.

Jantzen, G. M. (2001). Good sex: Beyond private pleasure. In P. Jung, M. Hunt, R. Balakrishnan (Eds.), *Good sex: Feminist perspectives from the world's religions* (pp. 3-14). New Brunswick: Rutgers University Press.

Keating, A. (2005). Shifting perspectives: 'Spiritual activism,' social transformation, and the politics of spirituality. In A. Keating (Ed.), *EntreMundos/AmongWorlds: New perspectives on Gloria Anzaldúa* (pp. 241-254). New York: Palgrave Macmillan.

Lara, I. (2006). *Decolonizing the sacred: Healing practices in the borderlands*. Manuscript in preparation.

León-Portilla, M. (1963). *Aztec thought and culture*. Norman: Oklahoma University Press.

López Austin, A. (1988). *The human body and ideology: Concepts of the ancient Nahua*. (T. Ortiz de Montellano & B. Ortiz de Montellano, Trans.). Salt Lake City: University of Utah Press.

Lorde, A. (1984). Uses of the erotic: The erotic as power. In *Sister outsider: Essays and speeches* (pp. 53-59). Trumansburg: The Crossing Press.

Marcos, S. (1991, December). Gender and moral precepts in ancient Mexico: Sahagun's texts. *Concilium: An International Review of Theology, 6*, 60-74.

Martínez, E. (1998). A word about the great terminology question. In *De colores means all of us: Latina views for a multi-colored century* (pp. 1-3). Cambridge: South End Press.

Pesquera, B., & Segura, D. (1998). 'It's her body, it's definitely her right:' Chicanas/Latinas and abortion. *Voces: A Journal of Chicana/Latina Studies 2*(2), 103-127.

Rodriguez, G. M. (2001). DeAlmas Latinas (the souls of Latina women): A psychospiritual culturally relevant group process. *Women & Therapy, 24*(3/4), 19-31.

Strasburger, V. C. (2000). Getting teenagers to say no to sex, drugs, and violence in the new millennium. *Medical Clinics of North America, 84*(4), 1-22.

Wiesner-Hanks, M. E. (2000). *Christianity and sexuality in the early modern world.* New York: Routledge.

Zavella, P. (2002). Talkin' sex: Chicanas and Mexicanas theorize about silences and sexual pleasures. In G. Arredondo et al. (Eds.), *Chicana feminisms: A critical reader* (pp. 228-253). Durham: Duke University Press.

Five Therapists' Personal and Professional Reflections and Integration

Sally D. Stabb
Debra Mollen
Carmen Cruz
Kelly Simonson
Avni Vyas
Karin H. Bruckner

SUMMARY. Women come to the therapeutic table with varying degrees of integration of sexuality and spirituality. Some have felt harmed by traditional religious interpretations and practices, others embrace these, and still others recreate and reclaim this integration in ways that are empowering and meaningful to them. Both the literature and the profession's guidelines have compelled us to begin with ourselves as women who are therapists. Five diverse women who are therapists share their own personal accounts of their sexuality and spirituality. Their experiences and identities run the gamut from keeping spirituality and sexuality distinctly separate to finding sacred meaning in the intersection.

Sally D. Stabb, PhD, and Debra Mollen, PhD, are affiliated with the Texas Woman's University Department of Psychology. Carmen Cruz, PsyD, is affiliated with the Florida Atlantic Counseling Center. Kelly Simonson, PhD, is affiliated with the Texas Woman's University Counseling Center. Avni Vyas, PhD, and Karin H. Bruckner, MA, LPC, are independent practitioners.

41

INTRODUCTION

We stand at an interesting point in time as therapists working with women's spiritual and sexual issues. Long strands of tradition, history, science, culture and change are in continuous flux and tension. Complexity is the rule, not the exception. We find juxtaposed conservative religious movements, new-age body-mind integration forces, and political and social agendas that are in stark debate about sexuality, sexual orientation, and the role of religion in women's lives. Our first responsibility is to know where we stand as therapists, as women ourselves in our collaborative effort to assist others in self-knowledge and in coming to places of peace with their own spirituality and sexuality.

Issues of religion, spirituality, and sexuality are routinely brought into therapy both as primary foci and as material surfaces throughout treatment, coupled with complex gender roles and gender socialization within religious and sociocultural contexts. Recent studies have demonstrated the importance a wide variety of clients place on discussing religious, spiritual, and sexual issues in therapy (Johnson & Hayes, 2003; Lease & Shulman, 2003; Morrow, 2003; Rose, Westefeld, & Ansely, 2001; Sherkat, 2002). Turner, Center, and Kiser (2004) remarked that because most people living in the United States have some degree of religious heritage and practice, it is incumbent upon therapists to explore these facets with their clients.

RELIGION, SPIRITUALITY AND SEXUALITY: FROM A CRITICAL PERSPECTIVE TO MEASURED RECONCILIATION

As a starting point, we as therapists must realize that the primary U.S. religious traditions of Christianity, Judaism, and Islam, coupled with the complex influences of gender, culture, and nation, have resulted in a degree of sexual oppression for many (Turner, Center, & Kiser, 2004). Recently illustrated examples include families of LGB individuals who cope with the religion/sexuality paradox by remaining silent and partially or wholly rejecting formal faith practices (Lease & Shulman, 2003), the rarely effective practice of conversion therapy (Morrow, 2003), experiences of self-hatred by Catholic lesbians (Walker, 2004), bias in blaming victims for rape by fundamentalist clergy (Sheldon & Parent, 2002), and the hesitance to disclose lesbian/bisexual identity when one has extremely religious parents (Mathy & Schillace, 2003).

Paradoxically, and simultaneously, others offer more positive interpretations of religious scripture and teachings. Spiritual exploration of sexuality can occur both inside and outside traditional religious organizations and offer clients and therapists unique areas to consider. Turner, Center, and Kiser (2004) noted that the overlap between sexuality and spirituality can engender a search for wholeness, harmony, meaning, connection, greater self-understanding, and mutual fulfillment. The possibilities for growth, purpose, and the melding together of these two critical aspects of humanity are seen by many as both attractive and attainable (Hutchins, 2002; Ullery, 2004; Yarhouse, 2005).

There is ample evidence in phenomenological accounts of how positive and powerful the intertwining of sexuality and spirituality can be. MacKnee's (2002) interviews with 10 individuals who reported "a profound event in which sexual and spiritual connection had occurred" (p. 236), noted a sense of wonder, emotional cleansing, a sense of God's presence evident, intense union, euphoria, transcendence, holistic involvement, blessing, ineffable mystery, and a sense of sacredness and worship. Aftereffects of transformation and relational healing, empowerment, passionate awareness, gratefulness, and gender equality were found. Well-established Eastern, Tantric practices have long demonstrated that connection with the spiritual can be a realizable and desirable goal of sex (Hutchins, 2002). Ullery (2004) emphasized that all sacred sex is embedded in meaning and value, and is never approached in a cavalier manner.

THE CURRENT PROJECT

What do these trends mean to us as women therapists hoping to assist other women in their own struggles around sex and spirituality? First, a clear call for starting with self-awareness as the very foundation for each therapist's clinical work was noted even in our very brief literature review. In addition to basic knowledge of both sexuality and core religious constructs, to know our own identities, biases, and intersections is the critical first step in sensitivity to diversity (APA, 2003). We hope that in sharing our backgrounds, others will have a powerful, first-hand account of how different each of us are as women, as spiritual, sexual, cultural beings ourselves. Our diversity is the diversity of our clients. Our willingness to know ourselves is a springboard on which all our interventions with the women who come to see us are based. What follows are five personal accounts of sexuality and spirituality from women who are therapists; we did not require a standard script or provide a set of guided questions, in an effort to best capture each women's unique experience and perspective.

AUTOBIOGRAPHICAL ACCOUNTS OF SPIRITUALITY AND SEXUALITY

Avni

I am a heterosexual, married female who crosses the "other" box when asked for my ethnicity as there exist no categories by which I can identify myself. While my origin, formal conditioning, and cultural upbringing are Indian, specifically within the Brahmin caste, I was born and raised in Africa as were my grandparents. However, I have lived in the west for most of my life, in part seeking good academic education.

I was raised in a culture with strong male dominance believing that women exist only to support men and serve all their needs. This is in sharp contrast with the education I received, especially in the later years, which placed a strong emphasis on diversity and women's issues. In spite of my formal education, I still have this strong undercurrent of catering to men, whether a husband, father, uncle, nephew, colleague, or boss. As a child, I worshipped my mother. Her stories, her mannerisms, her beliefs, her teachings, and her meaning of life were all etched in stone for me. While a man was indulged, a woman's role was likewise fulfilled, ensuring that she too would be happy.

The wealth of any family was measured by the number of children one had, especially boys. Oftentimes, there seemed to be a race to have as many boys as one could while those who did not have sons were pitied and condemned. This exemplifies the enduring values of the culture which have been upheld regardless of time, space, and education. The impact of culture is so strong that I can relate to and identify with characters in movies that portray life in very small villages in the 16th century or even identify with characters in folk songs that glorify gods like Rama who lived about 2500 years ago or Krishna who inhabited this planet almost 5000 years ago in India, a country that I have only visited as a tourist.

The strong dominance of the caste system was practiced in all the households in which I lived while growing up. Brahmins are supposed to be the highest caste, the caste that can do no wrong due to their birthright and can forgive the sins of others; they were the next best to god, seen as the primary communicators to all the gods. Yet, women were still women; they never measured up to men.

Sexuality was embedded within the day-to-day spiritual routine. That sexuality was based in spirituality was never a question. In fact it was hard to try to differentiate the two when I first reflected on the similarities between the two. While sex and spirituality went hand-in-hand, sex was never discussed directly, explicitly, or in a lustful form, but much more subtly or coyly. Sexual undertones were evident in folklore, in the god songs and prayers sung on daily basis, depicting how Krishna was teasing his *gopis* (female worshippers), or performing prayer routines to the *Shiva Lingum* (the male phallic symbol), or prayers for young brides to be fertile, or how young maidens could appease their men through adornments and the vivid colors of their outfits. In prayer rooms were erotic statues and Tantric (the spiritual merging of male and female sexual energies) images.

What is confusing and awkward is that while there were goddesses for almost all major dimensions of living, e.g., prosperity, wealth, knowledge, etc., the wife was not viewed in the same light. Women were basically trained as girls to take care of household functions, socialize, raise children, and indulge in so-called soft tasks such as knitting, embroidery, sewing, and painting. Girls cooked and put dishes away. They then graduated into harder tasks such as chopping veggies, making dough, sifting grains and flours, and still later making curries, rolling chappaties, making delicacies, and pickles. When the girl was of marriageable age and the would-be groom's family came to see her, she was required to make the meal and oftentimes the mother-in-law-to-be, who sat in another room, was able to determine the girl's ability to roll chappaties by the rhythm of the jangles of the girl's bracelets. She was a great candidate for marriage if she passed tests like these although they were both subtle and tricky.

Not only do I not cook well, but I dislike cooking. I cook just when necessary and can only prepare the basic foods. I'm not fussy. My husband, on the other hand, is a fine connoisseur. Yet, I would feel utterly responsible if he did not enjoy eating out and hated my food. He, of course, was raised like most men in our culture of not knowing most of the household chores. He can fix things around the house when he has time, but cannot cook, clean, or do most of the housework. Although my mother compelled me to be independent–and even with all my education and palpable courage–I feel guilty when my husband does not eat well. Yet, I consider myself a rebel, clearly a feminist, able to use my minority experiences and sensitivity in therapy.

My ongoing effort is to integrate my solid education in women's issues and the spiritual dimension of power of various goddesses vis-à-vis conditioning of a female within a Brahmin community as I continue to empower women in clinical settings. In therapy, my exposure to subtle sexual tones makes it easier for me to pick up subtle nuances, non-verbal messages, or chemistry that may exist between individuals. This also creates greater empathy and sensitivity to clients of mainstream as well as diverse backgrounds, and very often my clients provide feedback that they feel respected and find it easy to join with me. This heightened sensitivity of sexuality embedded in spirituality is perhaps the reason why I find it difficult to work with sexual perpetrators and have to refer them out.

In my role as a therapist, I continue to struggle with how religious beliefs dominate many of the decisions that my clients make. Many of my clients are very intelligent, seeking therapy for a range of issues from struggles with a mother-in-law to PTSD. I often catch myself competing with god as my clients and I try to resolve issues, or problem-solve when my clients' staunch religious beliefs and desires to abide by the "good book" far outweigh much of the assumed progress that has been achieved in therapy or what seems logical and rational to me. These are but some examples of my continuing struggle to integrate my multicultural sense of self as an effective feminist therapist working with issues of sexuality and spirituality.

Carmen

I was raised in the Catholic tradition, with more of a culturally Catholic practical experience than ascribing to the dogma of the faith. For example, we did not attend church every Sunday. We attended and participated at services for the holy holidays as well as family ritual events at church (e.g., baptisms, communions, confirmations, etc.). Within our Cuban culture, it is of utmost importance that one remains within the religion, regardless of spiritual practice. It is a membership that does not expire and something with which one is expected to continue identifying, almost regardless of practice.

What I learned about sexuality in my culture was twofold, which now I believe represents the intersection and reconciliation of immigrant women's struggle with defining themselves. On the one hand, from the older women in the culture I received the very traditional viewpoint of women's sexuality of suppression and *marianismo* (the term for the female counterpart of *machismo,* originating from the idyllic Virgin Mary, meaning sex role based behavior in which the woman is expected to suffer without complaining and to place the needs of her children, parents, and husband before her needs and desires). I also received more contemporary ideas from younger women in the culture allowing more freedom of expression, though not to the extent of Anglo women.

As a lesbian woman of color, I exist and manage a polycultural world with different rules, stereotypes, and expectations for each one. For instance, it seems that each cultural group with which I identify has unique developmental rules and expectations, as in being a "baby dyke" when one is coming out regardless of age in the lesbian culture, or that Latina women are often considered possessions to the men in their lives, the rule and stereotype of my Cuban identity.

I have struggled to feel fully at home with lesbians who are not Cubans and with Cubans who are not lesbians. I have wrestled with not feeling fully connected to both cultures and have found it difficult to find others who can understand my spiritual leanings. My belief now is that those with whom I emotionally connect, I share spiritual space.

Spirituality and sexuality are linked for me in multiple layers. First is recognition of the other person as someone to whom I am attracted, across spectrums of emotionality, physicality, and spirituality. It is a form of self-expression as well as the recognition that I feel somehow connected to the other person. The sense of feeling spiritual with someone does not necessarily have a traditional sexual component attached. There are many interactions that have a sense about them that others may not attribute to sexuality; however, my belief is that there is often a sexual and/or physical component to those interactions. For me, initial signs that can reflect a type of sexual connection include my heart beating faster, a heightened sense of awareness, tactile/tingling sensations, and visceral reactions, which can occur in friendships, romantic love, a collegial relationship, etc. The next step is how I interpret those feelings, both emotional and physical, and attach meaning to them. What is significant to me is the presence of connection and how I attach meaning to it.

The ability and opportunity to be connected to someone is a precious experience. The levels we allow ourselves to feel connected vary across our mood, sense of safety, ability of both parties, etc. When one shares oneself with another person, there is sacredness about it. There is a special and unique connection between two souls, which is where it transcends into the spiritual realm for me. When one has the experience of having this connection with one person to whom one is physically attracted, then it can culminate in the ultimate experience of sexuality, spirituality, and emotionality.

This same phenomena for me happens with music, and specifically my instrument, the drum. The connection I feel with my drum, my body, the earth, my soul, and those of others present when I play, is a very spiritual experience which I experience with my mind, body, and soul, encompassing sexuality. I once had a drum teacher who said "one has not fully experienced the drum if one did not play it in between one's legs, pushed up against one's crotch." I believe that the more one can let go, the more one can experience across dimensions of understanding and experience, including spirituality. This is all related to the ability to allow oneself not only to connect with others, but also truly experience vulnerability and the ability to be in the undefined, which spirituality sometimes is.

My spirituality has changed as I am no longer a practicing Catholic, yet continue to identify as a Catholic. Presently, I identify as a cultural Catholic since my Cuban culture is so indelibly imbedded in Catholicism and thus difficult to tease apart. One thing I enjoy from the Catholic faith and practice is the presence of ritual. I also participate in baptisms, communions, etc. of family members, and recite the traditional "Our Father" when recited in unity. This concept is similar to the identity of a cultural Jew versus a religious Jew. I practice more Earth-based spiritualities, specifically Native American traditions. These traditions allow for self-expression, regardless of identity. They recognize the power of women. They allow me to connect to the Earth, whose power is immense, as well as acknowledge my ancestry. These traditions are a better representation of how I see women, men, and sexuality, than in organized Western religions in which people are socialized to varying degrees to suppress their sexuality and emotionality. Western society raises women to suppress sexuality and much emotionality and trains men to suppress their emotionality and employ their sexuality. Native American and other Earth-based spiritual practices allow for more of an integration of both masculine and feminine qualities and thoughts.

What I do in therapy with women and men around issues of spirituality and sexuality, of course, depends on with what they are struggling and how it may be part of either one of these two facets of their lives. However, I usually find that people tend to enjoy talking about what they believe and essentially, that is what we do in therapy. Thus, in my practice, I tend to explore a person's belief system early on in therapy to gain further understanding of how they came about to be who they are, what they believe, why they act the way they act, and so on. In therapy I help clients explore how their experiences within their culture, religion, and family impacts what they believe today, hoping that increased self-awareness can then help with their struggles. So I recommend that therapists take the time with their clients, both male and female, and explore their beliefs. I have found that beginning with the construct of gender works well for many clients, as there is much material to examine. As each potential intersection and social location emerges, the therapist can explore how each part of clients' cultural identities, individually and collectively, may impact the client's current struggles and/or interpersonal relationships. Feminist theory posits that gender roles and socialization strongly contribute to a person's functioning in the world; therefore an exploration of beliefs is congruent with feminist therapy principles of practice.

Debra

I grew up in New Jersey in a Conservative Jewish home with my parents, two sisters, and brother. Like many Jewish Americans raised during the 1970s and 1980s, my exposure to Judaism was less religiously focused and more centered on the cultural experience of being a Jew. Well-assimilated in my working class Christian hometown, I embraced Jewish concepts, such as the values placed on intellectualism, questioning dogma, creating community, and repairing a damaged world, without knowing where these originated.

Regarding sexuality, I received a mix bag of messages and meanings which served to confuse me a great deal. On the one hand, I was raised with liberally-held ideas that I continue to embrace: the importance of reproductive freedom, access to abortion, support for lesbian and gay rights, and so on. Jewish teachings tend to view sex largely positively (albeit within the context of heterosexual marriage). Instead of equating sex with sin, I was taught that Jews view sex as essential to marriage, as a celebration of love, and that sex on the Sabbath was sanctified by G-d as a double *mitzvah* (good deed).

The inconsistencies and confusion that arose stemmed more from gender than from sex per se, and likely as much from the cultural zeitgeist of the era during which I was raised as from religious and spiritual messages. In its traditional practice, Judaism is a patriarchal faith, replete with sexist ideals and misogynistic inclinations. For example, as with many Western religions, G-d is nearly always referenced in the mascu-

line. In a traditional *minyan* (prayer circle), ten men are required to recite special prayers together. The traditional Jewish blessing that men
speak upon wakening, in which they praise G-d for not creating them as
women, has always seemed especially insulting to me. In my own family, my brother was more highly regarded than my sisters and I. He was
afforded more privileges, flexibility, and freedom than we were. Mean-
while, I remember painful and awkward discoveries as my body developed sexually at an alarming rate.

My Jewish identity entered a moratorium during my adolescence and
it was not until I was in my mid-20s and pursuing my Master's degree
that I was compelled to reexamine it in the bounds of a cross-cultural
psychology class. I grappled with the marriage of my internalized
anti-Semitism and the gifts I knew Judaism had afforded me. In the en-
suing years, I became intrigued by Native American practices and participated in a sweat lodge in 2002 in which I felt enriched and excited by
the connection I have always felt to the earth and its inhabitants. I found
the practice of calling in the directions of the Native American medicine
wheel among the most beautiful of all rituals and found joy in drum-
ming circles, smudging, and the quiet camaraderie I have witnessed in
these communities. Recently, I was made aware of the connection between Native American practices and Judaism and felt reassured of my
identification with each. When my husband and I married last year, we
combined our favorite rituals of each tradition in our wedding ceremony.

Currently, I see sexuality and spirituality along continua that often–but
not imperatively–overlap. I believe it is possible to embrace sexuality
for recreation and exploration without adding a spiritual element, and I
believe there are many devoutly spiritual people who abstain from sexual activity for a myriad of reasons. One of the benefits of having jour-
neyed a turbulent first third of my life is the intense amount of learning
I've done, admittedly some of it the hard way. Now, though, I see my
sexuality as intensely spiritual, as connecting me to my partner in the
most sacred of ways, and in turn, in connecting me to earth and animals
and ritual and others.

My experience as a therapist compels me to remain open and intrigued
by the many other ways people choose to integrate–or not–spirituality
and sexuality. I have been fortunate, in many ways, to have grown up as
a religious minority and to have had relationships and friendships with
people from many faiths and cultural groups. I recognize and celebrate
the different ways clients understand spirituality, practice or reject religion, and integrate or separate sexuality. My hope is that I draw on my

own experiences and understand myself deeply so that I might help others do the same.

Kelly

I was raised in northeastern Ohio by parents who were not especially religious themselves. I grew up middle-to-upper-middle class and was the youngest of three kids. As a family, we attended a local Presbyterian church for a few years mostly because my mother thought that education in Christianity was important culturally and as a way to connect with a community. I was not particularly interested in church and I had never felt any of the faith or any connection with a higher power that I imagined I was supposed to feel, so given latitude about religious education, I said no.

Since then, my views of religion have not changed much. I still have never felt a true connection with a higher power and I'm unsure if there is even a God. I have had some exposure to earth-based Pagan spiritual practices and find those more intriguing and more of a fit with me but not enough to continue to explore them on my own. I see spirituality as different from religion and feel I am a somewhat spiritual person though not religious. For me, religion has to do with a specific faith and its practices, dogma, and official leaders. Religion seems like something that is practiced in a particular way in a particular setting and feels much more narrow to me than does spirituality. I believe spirituality has more to do with one's faith (in God, in people, in nature) and less with a specific list of rules, regulations, and dogma. I believe spirituality can occur anytime, anywhere, and that it has as its essence a belief in the interconnection of all things and all people and is often more rooted in nature for me. It includes a sense of being connected to all other beings in this world and the security and comfort of this as well as the scariness of the vastness of this idea. It also includes a sense of karma and energy: that what you put into the world is then returned to you, that things happen for a reason even if that reason is not immediately apparent, and that putting positive energy into things often helps them materialize.

For me, spirituality and sexuality are two very separate things. Occasionally, I can feel a spiritual level of connection with another person while having sex, but this is relatively rare for me. It is much more common that I feel a human, physical and emotional connection with someone during sex, but it is rare that I would label this as spiritual. In some ways, I feel I may be missing out by not having this deeper connection, but in other ways, I feel lucky to be able to separate sexuality from spirituality and, in particular, from religion. Because the two have never had a connection for me and because my religious teachings were relatively short-lived and liberal, I don't feel I've had to work through as much baggage about sex. I see sex mostly as a positive thing that can be beautiful, fun, and about connecting through pleasuring someone you care about and pleasuring yourself. It can also be something that can be joyful and creative.

I have some hang-ups due to my socialization as a woman about worrying about being a "slut" if I have "too many" sexual partners, have sex "too soon," or enjoy it "too much," but age, experience, and my feminist friends and discussions have helped me challenge much of this thinking. I also think that not having sex and religion tied together has allowed me to develop much more liberal ideas about people in general, but especially around the issue of sexual orientation. I identified as heterosexual for years, but the more I learned about sexual continua of behavior, thoughts, fantasies and attractions, the more I opened myself up to the idea that love can come in any package. This led me to identifying myself as bisexual and being open to a loving connection with a person of either sex. This has allowed me to be a more powerful ally to other LGB people who have felt shamed by their religion and felt outcast.

My parents talked little about sexuality and tended to avoid the topic with me. I dated little in high school and was not sexually active. I was also overweight as a teenager (and still am a large woman) so I think this helped my parents to continue to avoid the topic of sexuality with me, as they misbelieved that big girls aren't sexual. Since high school, I've had to learn how to love and accept my body more at any size and shape and learn how to own my sexuality and sensuality within my body. For this, I mostly credit feminism. Feminist thought helped me feel stronger and more confident, care less about the outside package, and care more about the brains and heart on the inside. I also credit my mother for this because she and I have nearly identical bodies and I saw her explore her own sexuality and begin to approach and date men after my parents divorced, and she was seen as beautiful and desirable. My mother has served as a role model and offers me hope.

Additionally, more recently, I have begun a form of mind-body-spirit fitness called Nia that focuses on the joy of movement, body pleasure as opposed to pain, and that emphasizes individual expression of beauty and emotions. There is focus on the spirit through discussion of many Eastern concepts such as *chi* (our essential life-force), as well as encouraging people to express their own inner spirit and to use imagery to focus on transforming negative energy to positive energy in an aim toward healing. I have found this to be an empowering form of exercise that reinforces that beauty comes in many different packages and each of those packages can be sexy and sensual in their unique movements. This practice has increased my self-confidence as a woman and as a sexual being while also incorporating focus on spirituality.

As a therapist, I often see my own issues reflected in other women. I think women of all ages, shapes, and sizes have to work incredibly hard to love their bodies *as they are*. I have devoted myself to working in the area of improving body image for all people and for decreasing the prevalence of eating disorders. I think body image concerns are often incredibly detrimental to women's sexuality and can create major problems in relationships. When a woman does not feel comfortable in her body, how can she possibly relax and have sex, not to mention asking her partner to change something in order to increase her own pleasure? Sexuality issues are also very often linked to confidence, self-esteem, and assertiveness. The more confident a woman is in herself, the more beautiful and sexy she will seem and the more likely she will be able to enjoy sex and see it as a mutually pleasurable experience. For some women, having a greater spiritual connection with their partner or with a higher power may increase their self-confidence and self-esteem and, in this way, may positively contribute to their sense of sexuality.

Karin

I am a licensed therapist, researcher, and writer who practices from a family systems perspective. My clinical experience includes counseling for a public school district and employee assistance program, as well as private practice; my research has focused on women's anger and, more recently, the relationship between anger and sexuality. I am 49 years old and divorced, with three grown children. Spirituality has been an important part of my life since the age of 13, and so I have wrestled with issues of the sacred for over 35 years now. I've recently become engaged to a man who shares my dedication to spiritual growth, among many other things.

I believe that when I physically consummate a relationship with another, there are a number of experiences involved. Along with enjoying ourselves and developing an intense connection, we also play out and demonstrate in the physical realm the potential we have for a joyful and intense personal relationship with God. Sex is not only a celebration of love between two human beings, it is also the metaphor for the bliss of our spiritual union with the Ultimate Spirit. This means that each time we engage in the sexual act, there is a spiritual component involved that goes beyond our limited human souls and reaches into the divine. It's there for us to experience, but how often do we access it? How many of us seek God in such a place?

The implications of this perspective affect my spirituality and my sexuality on a day-to-day level. My faith must involve an intensely personal relationship with God if it is to accommodate the intimacy signified by sexual union. And my sexuality must span the gap we humans have placed between sensuality and holiness. Living this out means my choices and expectations are considered unique and are markedly different from those of the culture in which I live. For example, alongside my liberal, feminist perspective, I practice abstinence from sex outside of marriage. This view comes not from a legalistic adherence to religious laws, but rather from my desire to honor the mystery and miracle of how God relates to each human being and the expectations that places on us in this life.

I think the most important thread that ties spirituality and sexuality together is love. With this perspective, sex is more than just the fulfillment of a healthy human need, so much more than just a way to achieve physical release or experience pleasure. It is an exquisite means for expressing and receiving an exquisite love. So, too, our relationship with God goes far beyond a means for explaining our own existence, assuaging our guilt or quieting our fears. Our very essence, the stuff of which we are made, is a concrete expression of divine love, and we live in order to celebrate that love over and over again with every new day. Thus, out of divine love, we have been invited to dance with God in spiritual communion, and through sexual union we have a way to dance out this love with each other.

I haven't actually had the opportunity to address this relationship between sexuality and spirituality with a client. It's hard enough for most to dig down deep on just one of these topics, never mind both at the same time! When issues of sexuality surface, I try to create a space to view them within a larger context that includes spirituality, but am careful to follow a client's lead. The ways they choose to walk out their faith and the day-to-day decisions involving values and sexual behavior are their own. My belief is that we must take care of ourselves spiritually, just as we do physically, emotionally, and mentally; that we live our lives surrounded by and bathed in the love of a God who seeks to cherish each of us individually; and that the sexual act on its own and without a spiritual context falls far short of what we were created to be and to experience with each other. These concepts inform my therapeutic approach and seem to hold meaning for the realities my clients face.

REFLECTIONS AND DISCUSSION

What were your reactions to these five women therapists' stories? As the integrating author, I (Sally) am the one who knows all these women for varying years, the one who is not telling my story, but who is witness, like you, to their unique development. I am profoundly struck by the idiosyncrasies in each narrative and am keenly aware of the layered, complex unfolding of their identities over time. I simultaneously see intricately woven patterns throughout their stories and notice the vastly unique qualities of each.

All five women speak to their struggle to redefine self against sexist, gendered backgrounds, particularly the overvaluing of men and the traditional role of women in relation to men. Early gender role socialization messages are re-evaluated in the light of highly educated, feminist teachings, to which all five women have notably been drawn. Strands of discomfort around body image, acceptance of one's own sexuality, and choices in sexual behaviors linger. These struggles have merit, holding important life lessons that are likely to enhance each therapist's capacity for insight and empathy.

Another facet that deserves consideration is the way in which spirituality and sexuality are influenced by culture, nation, and family. Yankee, Latina, Hindi, or Heartland derived, the ways sexuality are made available to us as women and the ways it has been denied receive contemplation and reflection. Each woman finds components that suit her and ones that need revision, rejection, or reconciliation, within or outside of a spiritual context.

Of critical importance, these five women run the gamut in terms of linking spirituality and sexuality. On one hand, Kelly reports virtually no overlap in her lived experience of these two aspects of humanity, and is largely untroubled by this. We must be open to her and other women for whom this is the case, never trying to coerce an integration that doesn't resonate. At the other end of the spectrum, Karin's deeply enmeshed sense of the sexual and divine must be honored. Carmen and Debra have touched on this fusion as well, perhaps at a less consistent level, but with powerful emotion nonetheless. Avni speaks of the subtle interplay of sexuality in Hindi religious/cultural life that she experienced in Kenya, and continues to make sense of the integration of different cultural, spiritual, and national values about gender and sexuality.

Connection seems important and broadly construed for each woman, sometimes encompassing sexuality, sometimes spirituality, or neither–it can be in the context of friendship, music, or family for example. Contemporary views of women's development such as the Stone Center's Relational-Cultural Model (Jordan, 1997; Miller & Stiver, 1997), in which self evolves within relationships, fit well here. Mutual engagement, sensitivity, authenticity, a capacity for action, and process within relationships are cornerstones to this development and can be heard in each narrative. The pull for such connection may well provide for continuity across sexual, spiritual, and other domains in our clinical work, conceptually and pragmatically.

In getting to know these five women therapists, we hope readers join us in becoming sensitized to the many ways spirituality and sexuality present themselves in our lives so that we can continue these dialogues with each other and our clients. We strive to support our sisters in healing the hurts that some have experienced from the traditional religious interpretations of women's sexuality and to celebrate the ways that others have chosen to reconcile these for themselves. Above all, we remain mindful of the complexity of these intersections and honor the process of working through and the courage doing this takes.

REFERENCES

American Psychological Association (2003). Guidelines on multicultural education, training, research, practice, and organizational changes for psychologists. *American Psychologist, 58*, 377-402.

Hutchins, L. (2002). Bisexual women as emblematic sexual healers and the problematics of the embodied sacred whore. *Journal of Bisexuality. 2*(2-3), 205-226.

Johnson, C. V. & Hayes, J. A. (2003). Troubled spirits: Prevalence and predictors of religious and spiritual concerns among university students and counseling center clients. *Journal of Counseling Psychology, 50*, 409-419.

Jordan, J. V. (1997). *Women's growth in diversity: More writings from the Stone Center.* New York: Guildford.

Lease, S. H. & Shulman, J. L. (2003). A preliminary investigation of the role of religion for family members of lesbian, gay male, or bisexual male and female individuals. *Counseling & Values, 47*, 195-209.

MacKnee, C. M. (2002). Profound sexual and spiritual encounters among practicing Christians: A phenomenological analysis. *Journal of Psychology & Theology, 30*, 234-244.

Mathy, R. M. & Schillace, M. (2003). The impact of religiosity on lesbian and bisexual women's psychosexual development: Child maltreatment, suicide attempts, and self disclosure. *Journal of Psychology and Human Sexuality, 15*, 73-100.

Miller, J. B. & Stiver, I. P. (1997). *The healing connection: How women form relationships in therapy and in life.* Boston: Beacon Press.

Morrow, D. F. (2003). Cast into the wilderness: The impact of institutionalized religion on lesbians. *Journal of Lesbian Studies, 7*, 109-123.

Rose, E. M., Westefeld, J. S., & Ansely, T. N. (2001). Spiritual issues in counseling: Clients' beliefs and preferences. *Journal of Counseling Psychology, 48*, 61-71.

Sheldon, J. P. & Parent, S. L. (2002). Clergy's attitudes and attributions of blame toward female rape victims. *Violence Against Women. 8*, 233-256.

Sherkat, D. E. (2002). Sexuality and religious commitment in the United States: An empirical examination. *Journal for the Scientific Study of Religion. 41*, 313-323.

Turner, T. E., Center, H., & Kiser, J. D. (2004). Uniting spirituality and sexual counseling. *Family Journal: Counseling & Therapy for Couples & Families, 12*, 419-422.

Ullery, E. K. (2004). Consideration of a spiritual role in sex and sex therapy. *Family Journal: Counseling & Therapy for Couples & Families, 12*, 78-81.

Walker, G. (2004). Fragments from a journal: Reflections on celibacy and the role of women in the church. *Studies in Gender & Sexuality, 5*, 81-101.

Yarhouse, M. A. (2005). Constructive relationships between religion and the scientific study of sexuality. *Journal of Psychology & Christianity. 24*, 29-35.

Bridging the Divide:
Integrating Lesbian Identity
and Orthodox Judaism

Judith M. Glassgold

SUMMARY. Women who consider themselves traditional or conservative in the context of religious practice often experience tremendous
conflicts regarding the integration of same-sex emotional and sexual
feelings with their religion and spirituality. Current religious teachings
about homosexuality make this combination difficult as only heterosexual
sexuality within marriage is permitted in most orthodox faiths. Further, the way that spirituality and sexuality are conceptualized as oppos-
ing dichotomous categories (e.g., body vs. soul) presents women with a
framework where integration does not seem possible. Observant women
who come to psychotherapy often experience tremendous distress, guilt,
depression, and even suicidality due to the conflict between their sexual
feelings and religious doctrine. Relieving the distress, and resolving the
conflicts while honoring the emotional complexity of sexual feelings,
spirituality, and religious orthodoxy can present tremendous dilemmas for
the practitioner as well as the client. Using the example of psychotherapy

Judith M. Glassgold, PsyD, is a member of the Contributing Faculty, Graduate
School of Applied and Professional Psychology, Rutgers University, and is in Independent
Practice, Highland Park, NJ.

of an Orthodox Jewish woman who integrated same-sex desire into her life, this article describes psychotherapy process and alternative ways of viewing spirituality and sexuality that permit possible resolutions for clients.

INTRODUCTION

A client, Chaya, came to me with a question, "Am I a lesbian?" She admitted later that she had known the answer, but had been too terrified to ask the question aloud because she feared that any attempt to resolve the issue would divide her. She was an Orthodox Jew and her religious beliefs were experienced as essential to her being. She viewed her sexuality and spirituality as opposed to the other: being a lesbian was incompatible with being Orthodox, so being one meant the death of the other. Her assumptions about religious law presented her with an either/or dichotomy; thus, she could never be whole and no complete life was truly possible. This absolute, dichotomous framing of the dilemma kept her frozen in inaction and suffering.

The first issue in treatment, the question "Am I a lesbian," was in fact a question about possibility. For if, in her mind, it was not possible to be an Orthodox Jewish Lesbian, then she did not want to ask the question, the pain of awareness would be too great. Chaya would prefer to continue her experience of numbing depression and disassociated suffering, rather than deal with this sense of impossibility, which would create more pain. The problem was more: "If I cannot do it, why be it?" Being and doing were linked intrinsically for her; existence and possibility were one. If it is not possible, I do not wish to know. An interesting existential dilemma, "I can only be, if I can do."

The consequences of her religious and sexual orientation conflict appeared in very stark form: she feared being expelled from her Orthodox community and thus exiled. For her as well as many observant Jews, religious belief and community are inseparable. For some, religion is a set of relationships, a sense of belonging and family, as much as it is a belief system. Thus, to acknowledge her sexuality Chaya would have to face the potential loss of her spiritual community or figure out some way to avoid this loss. However, Chaya was clear she would never stop being Orthodox.

The first task I undertook was to point out this dichotomous conflict to Chaya, and to present the possibility that there was a way to transcend the dichotomy. I told her I was not sure what the solution would look like, but that is was worth exploring before she had to give up one of these two parts of her life. As I have family who are Orthodox Jews, I was able to discuss a female relative of mine, who though born in the 1920's had found a way to have a relationship with a woman in the context of Orthodox Judaism. I cautioned her that this relative's solution included many sacrifices and complexities, and took effort in both imagination and enactment, and might not fit Chaya's own needs. Chaya drew from this example the sense that she was not alone, and the knowledge that others had grappled with this problem.

Further, Chaya and I discussed in a very pragmatic way the issues she was going to have to address–she was married and had children–and I gave her the sense that it would take time to resolve these issues. I also told her that I did not know what the outcome would be. Chaya found this discussion helpful, and my expectation that treatment might take years rather than months, relieved her of the pressure of having to find a solution, and allowed her to explore her emotions. Further, my framing of these issues as extraordinarily complex validated her struggles with these issues.

FORMULATION:
DEVELOPMENT, SELF AND SEXUAL ORIENTATION

Each person evolves within a particular historical, social, psychological, religious, emotional, cognitive, and intellectual context. Their religious beliefs and emotional, sexual, and psychological lives are intertwined. Attempting to change or remove the spiritual beliefs or change Chaya's emotional and sexual expression would have done a disservice to this woman and distorted the problem (see Espín, 2005). In addition, the client's psychodynamics, as well as the present-day religious and cultural contexts played an important role in the evolution and expression of Chaya's religious and sexual potential. My approach integrated principles of feminist therapy, such as empowerment, modern theories of the psychology of women focused on connection and relationship (Gilligan, 1984; Jordan, J. V., Kaplan, A. G., Miller, J. M., Stiver, I. P., Surrey, J. L., 1991), psychodynamic theories, trauma theory, and multicultural theories that acknowledge multiple facets of identity.

Chaya had experienced both severe emotional neglect from her parents and physical abuse from an older brother. To cope with emotional and physical abuse as well as neglect, Chaya had learned to lose touch with her feelings through disassociative experiences. This way of surviving her family served as a means of interacting with the world, and integrating the stages of personal and sexual development of childhood, adolescent, and adulthood. Thus, she had dealt with her sexual orientation in a manner that was consistent with her approach to other problems: detachment, denial, and disassociation.

Chaya found her situation particularly challenging, and therapy difficult, as she could not experience certain painful emotions and memories without disassociation. She had no knowledge of what comfort or soothing felt like. Her disassociative defenses prevented her from being able to remain focused on her emotions in the present moment. This emotional disconnection prevented Chaya from completely understanding her life, which then limited her ability to develop wholeness, integrity, and ultimately agency. The life decisions that Chaya faced demanded very difficult decisions. In order to make these decisions, Chaya would have to be able to tolerate and process painful emotions. In my clinical judgment, this process was impeded by the disassociative defenses, so that treatment would first have to address this aspect of her psychodynamics. Thus, the early part of therapy focused on her learning how to bear her feelings and to soothe herself without disassociating.

It is my clinical observation, that those individuals who have had difficult or traumatic family lives, often address sexual orientation later in life after the traumatic difficulties have been somewhat resolved. Chaya fit this pattern. Her childhood and adolescence were focused only on emotional survival. In her adolescence, Chaya's sexual behavior was with men, but not out of sexual desire or erotic needs. She recounted a complete absence of sexual feelings or arousal. She was hungry for emotional contact of any sort, lacking that in her family. She discovered that men were willing to pay attention to her and make her feel special, if she would have a sexual relationship with them. These relationships were not sexually pleasurable and were often troubling and hurtful. Unfortunately, although she sought acknowledgment of her self, these hurtful relationships replicated the lack of recognition, validation, and emotional abuse of her family.

Chaya married a man she felt no desire for. She cared about him a great deal and thought that he would make a good husband. She asked family members about this lack of sexual interest on her part, and was told that erotic interest was not that important in a long-term marriage.

She married her husband and saw sex as one of her obligations. He noticed the disparity of their feelings and her complete lack of passion or interest in sex, so as a couple they consulted a few therapists. Therapy did little to change the problem and no therapist inquired about sexual orientation issues, probably not expecting this in an Orthodox couple. Chaya with her history of deprivation, had few expectations about desire and did not see this as an issue, nor did she comprehend how completely physically or emotionally unaroused she was.

Despite their sexual issues, her husband was a kind and loving man, who treated Chaya better than she had ever been treated. They created a loving family and parented well together. She raised her children much differently than she herself had been raised, not only in a religious sense, but also in the level of child-centeredness, emotional attunement, and protection. Her marriage was emotionally healing, and may have helped her resolve some of her intrapsychic issues, so that now she was at a stage to explore her sexuality.

THERAPY: SELF AND RELIGION

As her ability to tolerate her feelings increased, Chaya could begin to grapple with the central dilemma that had brought her to treatment, her sexual orientation, and religion. Exploring the possibility of whether there could be a combination intrigued her. This was not an option she envisioned, the situation of many people of conservative faith (Haldeman, 2004). However, the fact that this dilemma was so difficult for her cannot be separated from her intrapsychic issues. The intrapsychic issues were important to explore first, as to lay a foundation, where she could tolerate the emotions that would emerge as her life evolved.

One of the dilemmas some religiously committed individuals and practitioners often address is changing sexual orientation through psychological treatments (Gonsiorek, 2004; Haldeman, 2004). As Chaya realized that she was a lesbian, she had to confront the reality that her marriage and her lesbian identity did not appear compatible. Bearing that loss, and the pain she would cause her husband and children were extraordinarily difficult, and she vacillated between avoidance, denial, and disassociation. As part of her attempting to address this conflict, and under pressure from some elements of her Orthodox religion, she asked if her sexual orientation could be changed through sexual orientation conversion therapy. I told her I did not perform such treatment for a variety of reasons, primarily lack of efficacy and ethics (see Shroeder & Shidlo, 2001 among others). Instead, we dealt with the emotions raised by this dilemma through my empathic understanding of her suffering. Confronting the tragic in life is an important part of all psychological treatment, especially in cases when someone is not who they would wish to be ideally. Further, facing what appear to be impossible choices must be emotionally confronted and grieved before any other resolution can be found.

Further, I invited Chaya, as an educated professional, to read the psychological literature on sexual orientation conversion therapy and we discussed her options. I invited her to consult with a conversion therapist if she wished, and discuss the results with me and remain in therapy. She did meet with an Orthodox Rabbi who had received some psychology training who offered conversion therapy based on a formulation that lesbianism was a developmental arrest. After meeting with him once, she decided not to pursue this treatment as he saw her problems through the view of old stereotypes about lesbianism, unresolved attachments to mother. His model of sexuality and sexual orientation felt to her to be full of odd psychobabble, and simply pathologized her feelings. She eventually learned to accept her sexuality and view it positively through empathic acceptance by me of all her feelings.

I believe that respecting her choices, while showing compassion for her suffering was essential. Further, I avoided presenting an either/or dilemma in our relationship: either accept or change her sexuality. I provided individual treatment while Chaya at different times tried marriage therapy as she tried to avoid ending her marriage, which had been the best relationship she had had to that point. My constancy and acceptance of her ambivalence was essential. She needed–for her own sense of integrity to her husband, children, and religion–to feel as though she had done everything to save the relationship. However, she and her husband discovered that they could not integrate their different sexual and emotional needs into a relationship and they eventually separated and divorced.

RELIGIOUS ISSUES

Chaya, as with many women, had to first discover her own self and feelings and then re-examine religious teachings to find out how to integrate her emotions, feelings, and behaviors within Orthodox traditions and law. For each individual, the specific meaning and importance of religion has to be explored. Often this exploration can benefit from a lifespan perspective, as with other aspects of identity, religious and spiritual beliefs evolve over time. Chaya's religious beliefs were an important alternative to her sense of aloneness in her family of origin. Raised within the Conservative Jewish tradition, Chaya discovered Orthodox Judaism in college and converted during those years. As some research has shown, many women find Judaism an important source of sustenance in the process of identity formation and religion can provide a means of well-being (Goldberg & O'Brien, 2005). Chaya found the spiritual authenticity of Orthodoxy refreshing.

Perhaps, more important was the strong community; the connections of care and concern and the sense of responsibility for each other's welfare was profoundly important to her. Thus, an important part of psychotherapy was exploring what was important to Chaya about her religious and spiritual beliefs and traditions. The personal experience of religion is unique and clarifying an individual's understanding of their spiritual priorities is essential. There is no one way to be Orthodox, and though perhaps subtle, these differences are important.

However, Chaya's beliefs were not respected by her family and caused separation and conflict within her family. This reaction mirrored earlier unempathic experiences with her family, especially her mother. As I am less devout than Chaya, which was obvious to her from the beginning from various signs such as dress, speech, and other aspects of self-presentation, it was important that I model a different means of interacting with her than her family of origin by respecting her religious beliefs and being open to acknowledging them and discussing our differences. Further, I admitted my own limitations, as did she, about the actual religious prohibition regarding female homosexuality in Orthodox Judaism. Here she had very little guidance from religious leaders, as they were fundamentally unfamiliar with lesbian sexuality and behaviors. Chaya found a community of information and support over the Internet and through other organizations with whom she could sometimes meet or correspond. This community of women by interpreting Talmud on their own or with help from sympathetic Rabbis (Friedman, 2004) struggled to make sense of their lives. Modern Orthodox Judaism offers flexibility through its attention to individual cases and application of law to individual dilemmas, allowing some flexibility within the tradition and options for women to study. Therefore, I encouraged her to study and find others who were more knowledgeable and bring what she had learned back into our work.

Judaism is based on scholarship, interpretation, and application of law. Chaya read widely and consulted many sources, including speaking to a wide number of Rabbis of a broad range of beliefs. The initial problem for Chaya and other women I have worked with are the philosophical assumptions about sexuality found in western religions. These assumptions about sexuality and spirituality do not match many women's emotions or their experience of sexuality, which incorporates love and spirituality. Further, traditional religious beliefs often present sexuality and emotions as separate. Thus, issues of connection, community, love, and companionship are not part of the framing of sexuality, which is of the body and identified as lust. As most western religions frame the appropriate place of sexuality within a religiously sanctioned heterosexual marriage, other forms of sexual expression are seen as impure or forbidden, whether activities, objects, or emotions. However, strong emotional ties between women are represented in religious texts, such as the Book of Ruth, and are interpreted positively. This contradiction presents problems for women as well as potential solutions.

Female sexuality in Orthodox Judaism is complex, and the primary principle is obedience to law, governed by the Talmud (first 10 books of the Old Testament), as well as interpretations of law by Rabbinic scholars. Those texts are referred to by modern-day scholars in interpreting the correct behavioral act. Feelings are generally not prohibited, unless resulting in an act. Much of what is written about female sexuality is not from actual experiences, but what is observable by men or assumed by them (Biale, 1984, p. 196); thus, it is removed from the concerns of daily life. Importantly, the standard for what is sex is male-initiated genital intercourse.

Female sexuality is seen as passive, not active (Biale, 1984, p. 122). Limitations are placed on sexual expression, it is to be within heterosexual marriage, and both behaviors and frequency are regulated (Biale, 1984, pp. 121-146). Sexual pleasure is acknowledged in women, which is important, but depending on the interpreter subject to regulations and limitations (Biale, 1984, p. 137). Modesty laws, for both men and women, are related to sexuality and define sexuality as purely based in the body.

Lesbian sexuality is not envisioned, thus not proscribed in Hebrew versions of Leviticus (unlike certain male sexual behaviors with another man (Leviticus 18:22 see Fox, 1983; Biale, 1984, pp. 192-197). The debate in Rabbinic texts is whether lesbian acts are actually sex, as what is traditionally defined as sex (male-female genital intercourse) does not occur (Biale, 1984, pp. 196-97). If certain erotic acts between women are not defined as sex, their legal status changes, these behaviors are deemed licentiousness and have fewer sanctions. However, these behaviors are interpreted by some as following the traditions of another culture or religion and therefore disobedience (Leviticus 18:3 "obeying the laws of Egypt" as in Fox, 1983, as interpreted by Maimodes, see Biale, 1984, pp. 195-196) and thus punished as such. However, not defining lesbian sexual behaviors as sex moves it to another area of discourse.[1]

Ironically, this invisibility of women in the Talmud and the definition of lesbian "non"-sexuality presented Chaya with possibilities. Placing lesbian sexual behavior as outside of sexuality, allowed her to avoid a complete prohibition: it was thus not governed by laws regarding sexuality. Without relevant precedent and without an accurate description of women's sexuality, Chaya felt freer to create her own vision based on the totality of Jewish principles, many of which are extremely humanistic. Chaya's own solution and understanding is unique to her, and focused on the interconnections of Jewish laws on a variety of topics (modesty, sexuality, marriage, women's concerns, suffering) as well as integrating modern science and psychology. She thus felt that her sexual orientation was unchangeable, basic to her essence, and the suffering she experienced when unable to be herself validated this. However, as Judaism is about law and regulation, she felt she had to make decisions regarding rules that regulated women's lives. Thus, she did not attend the mikvah (ritual bath) after menstruating, as she would not be engaging in what was defined as sexual behavior, and she did not believe that she could marry within the Jewish tradition, as a lesbian relationship could not be defined within the confines of Jewish law on marriage.

As a great deal of the importance of her religion was in its community, Chaya had to come out to her closest friends and strategize on how to maintain her ties within her community. Over a long period, she strategically came out to her closest friends, and fortunately, her community was liberal for an Orthodox community and her friendship network did not reject her when she came out. Managing disclosure and openness in her community were complex issues and had to be made pragmatically. Being able to be accepted by her community was so important and was crucial to her integration of religion and sexuality.

Chaya's sense of her self evolved to include a very different sense of self-respect and self-esteem. This culminated in her going to her Rabbi and informing him of her sexual orientation, asking to remain in the community to raise her children, and negotiating around issues of disclosure. She did not ask for his approval, and explicitly said that. Chaya takes her current partner (Jewish, but not Orthodox) to services and community events. She has sought inclusion, and has been able to achieve that, not in an absolute sense, but in a relative one, which has still allowed her enough autonomy to feel comfortable. She has discussed this issue with her children and they are comfortable with her and continue to be raised Orthodox. Chaya also participates in a Gay and Lesbian Jewish (non-Orthodox) community group and an Orthodox Lesbian women's online community. These relationships form an important network for her of social support, without having to rely on one community for all her emotional resources.

Importantly, I did not judge or evaluate her religious choices. She educated me to her decisions and her rationale, and as a psychologist, I feel I am not in the position to lead on those issues. Those who are Orthodox might have criticized her interpretation of law, but again, I felt that in a treatment that valued autonomy, those decisions were not mine to judge. Understanding where she had come from, I made great efforts to offer acknowledgement, respect, and self-determination. I made explicit steps to communicate that she was entitled to respect even when we disagreed.

NEW DIRECTIONS

The work with Chaya raises additional questions about the underlying assumptions that are embedded in views of sexuality and spirituality. For many religiously orthodox women, many of the conceptualizations underlying these concepts are both foreign and limiting. The Jewish definition of sexuality focuses on men and acts committed by men. Behaviors of women are different and unimagined. This presents women who are devout with a dilemma; they are seeking a way to integrate sexuality and spirituality, they are seeking guidance that makes sense of their emotions, but the existing models provide none. As most women experience their sexuality as an extension of emotional bonds, the rules of law are in many ways irrelevant. Other ways of conceptualizing sexuality, through intimacy, love, companionship, community, integrity, self-awareness, though present in small ways in some religions, has been made invisible over the generations leaving women few options: to be sexual in the way religion defines it (which can bear no resemblance to their feelings) or to have no sexuality at all.

Traditional models of spirituality are similarly unfamiliar to women. Most religions present themselves and their doctrines as truth, separate from context, and as unchanging over time. This, too, decontextualizes religion and separates it from the lived individual life. Some religions focus on absolute principles that do not advocate contextual moral decision-making, which is more similar to women's frameworks of connection and morality focusing on an individual's life situation (Gilligan, 1982). Most orthodox or fundamentalist religions focus more on morality that is separate from daily life struggles and based on rigid absolutes. Further, human development, including spiritual development, such as cognitive and emotional growth throughout lifespan, is minimized in orthodox belief systems; even the cognitive elements of belief are not seen as changing over the lifespan. If religious creed is absolute and unchanging, and morality is black/white, the individual has no role in shaping meaning, and then is left with a dichotomous option "believe or not believe."

Focusing on models of sexuality and spirituality that are more closely tied to women's realities provides far more alternatives for all women. Very few in mental health have attempted to integrate what we know about the psychology of women and other aspects of ethnic and racial diversity, and sexuality and spirituality in their discussions of orthodox or conservative views (Milville & Ferguson, 2004). Alternate views could focus far more on emotional concerns rather than those of the body. One specific goal should be reframing sexuality as possessing many components, where love, emotion, and connection rather than impersonal, decontextualized lust is essential to match women's (and many men's) realities. This vision is more consistent with the emotional realities of spirituality, which contains a sense of connectedness, whether to a divine essence, community, tradition, people, etc. as well as a composed of faith and love. Spirituality, as well, is far more complex and is often intertwined with personality, values, community, family ties, faith, love, and may evolve as all aspects of personality.

Audre Lorde (1984) in her essay: "Uses of the erotic: The erotic as power" proposes a totally different view of the erotic that takes into consideration women's realities and reframes the erotic: "The erotic is a resource within each of us that lies in a deeply female and spiritual plane, firmly rooted in the power of our unexpressed or unrecognized feeling" (Lorde, 1984, p. 53). Lorde goes on to define the erotic as a connection: "The sharing of joy, whether physical, emotional, psychic, or intellectual, forms a bridge between the sharers which can be the basis for understanding much of what is not shared between them, and lessens the threat of their difference" (Lorde, 1984, p. 54). The erotic is the capacity for joy, "the life-force once recognized of women; of that creative energy empowered (Lorde, 1984, p. 55). Such a concept emphasizes the integration of the spiritual with the erotic, the erotic as a source of inner power and joy as well as a means of connecting intimately with another. There are many other visions of both spirituality and sexuality more rooted in women's lives that provide both traditional and more modern women other ways to experience and integrate their emotions and beliefs.

For psychotherapists, being able to open up the possibility of other models can open up possibilities for treatment. Sexuality and spirituality are narratives, which women explore and rewrite. Sexuality and spirituality do not have to be seen as predetermined essences, which just reinforces the dichotomies, but as issues that go through a profound developmental journey. Although a set of beliefs can be "ageless," individual spirituality is a deeply felt personal creation with varied meanings, emotional valence, behaviors, much like other forms of identity.

For many women identity is not as in traditional western, Cartesian thought, "I think therefore I am." Rather identity is a set of relationships, connections to people, affiliations, constructs. Identity facilitates relationships and connections, but is not an essence in itself. Chaya's dilemma was that she feared her sexuality would sever one set of very valued relationships, connections, and communities. Instead, her community ties were maintained and new communities (Lesbian and Gay) and intimate partners were added.

Of course, there is the relationship to the self, a relationship that evolves over time. As with all relationships, identity, evolves, grows over time and ends up transformed. This is an expansion to, but perhaps different from, the concept of fluidity, which is commonly used in the context of describing women's sexual orientation (Golden, 1987). Fluidity literally means subject to change or movement. However, this word does not describe the nature of change, the meaning that is embedded in women's lives, and does not relate to the psychic depth of women's evolution. For those women who are spiritually committed, identities can be open, not a predetermined endpoint, fluid in the sense that they can change. But rather than randomly changing, identities part of the process of development, maturity, and evolving erotic potentials and spiritual beliefs, and practices. Sexuality or spirituality should not be subject to external pressures or inauthentic models that reflect oppression, privilege and culturally bound constructs (Espín, 2005; Milville & Ferguson, 2004) or artificial dichotomies (Phillips, 2004).

CONCLUSION

Chaya told me in our last session that the some of the most important things she learned in therapy (other than addressing her sexual orientation) were about human dignity and the development of what she considered was her own integrity. The concept of human dignity we defined was to know and ask for recognition for her needs. This was a fundamental premise of treatment, but also reflected a balance between her need for religious community, obedience to laws she felt were fundamental, ties to a community of ancient faith, and need for love, companionship, spiritual certainty, and family.

Orthodox Judaism emphasizes obedience to law and thus for her in particular the dilemma of submission versus autonomy was particularly salient. However, this was not a dichotomous opposite, and an exploration of the meaning of sexuality, self, and law resolved the breach. This did not mean terminating her relationship to her religion. She understood her own sexuality in different ways, outside of the pre-existing categories, and with a broader understanding of how her own sexuality and psyche were intertwined. She could not separate her sexual orientation from her self, as she could not leave her religion. However, by gaining a greater sense of integrity, accepting her feelings, and understanding her sexuality better, she integrated Lesbian sexuality into her religious life. The categories and conceptualizations of sexuality she inherited from society and her religion were unhelpful in this regard, and models closer to the reality of women's emotional lives were much more helpful. However, fortunately in her case, the essence of her religion was not its conceptualization of sexuality, but rather her relationship to God and desire to hold herself true to fundamental precepts.

Psychotherapists who grapple with traditional and orthodox religious clients are often faced with situations that seem irresolvable. However, this is often due to the psychotherapist's acceptance of existing frameworks or assumptions about religion, spirituality, and sexuality. Most models of psychotherapy, as well as sexuality and spirituality, have too long ignored women's perspectives and realities, compounding the dilemmas for women. Focusing on the strength of psychotherapy, which understands and client autonomy, refocuses therapy on its true aims, allowing someone to explore their life and learn to bear what seems unbearable in an imperfect world. Psychotherapy can be a place to gain a sense of wholeness that includes spiritual and religious integrity and greater belief, not by trying to determine the content of those beliefs, but rather aiding the individual in their own process of exploration.

NOTE

1. For a more detailed account of this issue, see *Wrestling with God and men: Homosexuality in the Jewish tradition*, Rabbi Steven Greenberg and *Women and Jewish Law*, Rachel Biale.

REFERENCES

Biale, R. (1984). *Women and Jewish law: The essential texts, their history, and their relevance for today*. NY: Schoken Books.

Espín, O. (2005, January). *The age of the cookie cutter has passed: Contradictions in identity at the core of therapeutic intervention*. Invited Address: National Multicultural Summit, Los Angeles, CA. Retrieved June 3, 2005 from APA Division 44 website: http://www.apa.org/divisions/div44/olivia.htm

Fox, E. (1983). (Trans). *The Five Books of Moses*. The Schoken Bible, Vol 1. NY: Schocken Press.

Friedman, S. (2004). *Wrestling with God and men: homosexuality in the Jewish tradition*. Madison, WI: University of Wisconsin.

Gilligan, C. (1984). *In a different voice: Psychological theory and women's development*. Cambridge, MA: Harvard.

Goldberg, J. J. & O'Brien, K. M. (2005). Jewish women's psychological well-being: The role of attachment, separation, and Jewish identity. *Psychology of Women Quarterly, 29*, 197-206.

Golden, C. (1987). Diversity and variability in women's sexual identities. In Boston Lesbian Psychologies Collective (Eds.), *Lesbian Psychologies: Explorations and Challenges* (pp. 18-34). Urbana, IL: University of Illinois.

Gonsiorek, J. C. (2004). Reflections from the Conversion Therapy Battlefield. *The Counseling Psychologist, 32*, 750-759.

Haldeman, D. C. (2004). When Sexual and Religious Orientation Collide: Considerations in Working with Conflicted Same-Sex Attracted Male Clients. *The Counseling Psychologist, 32*, 691-715.

Lorde, A. (1984). *Sister/Outsider*. NY: The Crossing Press. Trumansburg, NY: The Crossing Press.

Jordan, J. V., Kaplan, A. G., Miller, J. M., Stiver, I. P., Surrey, J. L. (1991). *Women's growth in connection: Writings from the Stone Center*. NY: Guilford Press.

Milville, M. L. & Ferguson, A. D. (2004). Impossible "Choices": Identity and Values at a Crossroads. *The Counseling Psychologist, 32*, 760-770.

Phillips, J. C. (2004). A Welcome Addition to the Literature: Nonpolarized Approaches to Sexual Orientation and Religiosity. *The Counseling Psychologist, 32*, 771-777.

Schroeder, M. & Shidlo, A. (2001). Ethical Issues in Sexual Orientation Conversion Therapies: An empirical study of consumers. *Journal of Gay and Lesbian Psychotherapy, 5*(3/4), 131-166.

What's Faith Got to Do with It? The Role of Spirituality and Religion in Lesbian and Bisexual Women's Sexual Satisfaction

Brandy L. Smith

Sharon G. Horne

SUMMARY. This study examined the role of faith, both religion and spirituality, on the sexual satisfaction of lesbian/queer and bisexual women (n = 318). A hierarchical regression was used to determine the potential influence of religion and spirituality above and beyond the variance explained by three background variables (i.e., age, sexual orientation, living with partner status). While religion did not significantly contribute to women's reports of sexual satisfaction, results indicated that both living with a partner and spirituality had a significant positive relationship with sexual satisfaction. In particular, two aspects of spirituality (spiritual freedom and connectedness) were strong predictors of sexual satisfaction.

Brandy Smith, PhD, teaches Clinical Psychology at the University of Memphis. Sharon G. Horne is Associate Professor, University of Memphis, Memphis, TN.

INTRODUCTION

Faith is an important part of many people's lives. It has been linked to helping people fight disease and cope more effectively if they suffer from a disease (Powell, Shahabi, & Thoresen, 2003), as well as maintain positive mental health (e.g., Koenig, 1998; Ventis, 1995; Worthington et al., 1996). Not only is increased faith associated with psychological well-being (Levin, Markides, & Ray, 1996), it also plays a role in the reduction of depressive symptomatology (Ellison, 1995) and the instillation of hope during stress (Ross, 1990).

The term *faith* is used in the title and throughout this paper to incorporate both spiritual and religious experiences. These two experiences are often viewed as two distinct constructs with spirituality defined as a person's individual connection with a faith and religion defined as the framework in which one practices his or her faith (Miller & Thoresen, 2003). Although spirituality and religion are two separate constructs and frequently serve different purposes in people's lives, they are both important to one's sense of connection to a higher being or purpose and can be combined in that sense. In instances when both aspects of connection are referenced, the term *faith* is used, but when the separate constructs are referenced, *spirituality* or *religion* will be used appropriately. That distinction will be particularly relevant for this study because the potential influences of both religion and spirituality were explored for their relationship to sexual satisfaction.

The relationship between gay, lesbian, and bisexual (GLB) persons and faith has been less clear than the relationship of heterosexual persons and faith. Many GLB individuals have experienced conflict between their faith and sexual orientation and have faced condemnation, rejection, and other disaffirming beliefs and practices towards GLB persons on behalf of organized religion (e.g., Barrett & Barzan, 1996; Schuck & Liddle, 2001). In addition, many GLB individuals have grown up in disaffirming religious environments and must reconcile their sexual orientation with their religious beliefs, which can be a very daunting task (e.g., Davidson, 2000). Morrow (2003) described the conflict that many lesbians experience with religion, particularly in Christian faiths, including such experiences as sexism, heterosexism, and harmful Biblical interpretations of female same-sex sexuality. Such research supports the findings of other research, which has shown that GLB persons frequently leave their faith group when its beliefs and/or practices conflict with their sexual orientation (e.g., Manley & Horne, 2003; Schuck & Liddle, 2001).

Despite the common occurrence of conflict between faith and sexual orientation, current research has shown that many GLB people do experience and enjoy a faith connection (e.g., Davidson, 2000; Smith & Horne, in press; Yip, 2002) and that participation in GLB-affirming faith communities has been shown to relate to psychological well-being and spirituality among GLB individuals (Lease, Horne, & Noffsinger-Frazier, in press). In addition, even though many GLB persons do leave their faith, they often leave and find another, more affirming faith so that they can maintain a faith connection (Lease & Horne, 2002; Yip, 2000). Another alternative that GLB persons appear to take once leaving an organized religion is to identify themselves as "spiritual" instead of religious (Schuck & Liddle, 2001). Consequently, many GLB individuals rate spirituality as more important in comparison to religion (e.g., Lee & Busto, 1991). Such research elucidates the need to include spirituality in addition to religion, which might be even more important when working with GLB persons and faith. In conclusion, despite negative experiences and associations for GLB persons with religion, research has found that GLB individuals do report faith affiliations (e.g., Davidson, 2000; Manley & Horne, 2003; Schuck & Liddle, 2001; Yip, 2002) and that those GLB individuals who participate in GLB affirmative faith groups report positive gains and experiences in terms of psychological health and spirituality (Lease, Horne, & Noffsinger-Frazier, in press).

As the benefits of faith have received attention in the field of psychology, the role of faith in therapy has evolved. Faith has historically been a topic that was not directly or explicitly included in the field of counseling psychology (Sue et al., 1999). However, that trend has changed in more recent years, particularly as therapists realized the important role faith plays in many clients lives, despite the lack of attention it was receiving in therapy (Rose, Westefeld, & Ansely, 2001). In an effort to work with clients in a more holistic manner, the field has begun to more thoroughly investigate the influence of faith.

Similar to faith, religion, and spirituality, sexual satisfaction is another important part of people's lives that has received scant attention within the psychology field. Allina (2001) noted that research in this area has developed within a medical model that does not recognize the full scope of women's sexuality. In addition, if the research on women's sexuality is not presented from a medical perspective, it frequently focuses on the more romantic, emotional components of women's sexuality, such as emotional intimacy and partner attractiveness (Howard, 1988; Sprecher, 2002); this is especially true for research on lesbian women's sexuality (Hurlbert & Apt, 1993; Rose, 1996). Women's sexuality, in particular, has been neglected within medical and psychological fields due to the prizing of male sexuality and historical misrepresentations of women's reproductive and sexual desires and constructions (Tiefer, 2001). Part of this stems from traditional gender stereotyping of women as less sexual than men, and when they are considered to have sexual agency, it is often conceptualized as greater investment in the emotional aspects of sexual relationships than men (e.g., Howard, 1988; Peplau, 2003; Sprecher, 2002).

Sexuality research has focused primarily on the experiences of heterosexual persons (e.g., Byers & Demmons, 1999; Deeks & McCabe, 2001; Dunn, Croft, & Hackett, 2000; Hurlbert, 1991; Sprecher, 2002; Young et al., 2000). Although there has been some sexuality research with gay and lesbian persons in recent years (e.g., Dupras, 1994; Meyer & Dean, 1994; Peplau & Garnets, 2000; Williamson, 2000), none has explored the role of religion and spirituality. This project aims to fill some of the gaps in sexuality research by investigating the experiences of lesbian and bisexual women.

In addition, research to date has not explored the separate but inter-related constructs of religion and spirituality with respect to sexual satisfaction. For example, it is unknown whether women who attend faith services and consider themselves religious, experience some benefits in their sexual experience. Similarly, women who report a strong sense of spirituality may also be more likely to be sexually satisfied. Therefore, this study investigated religion and spirituality separately for their relationship to sexual satisfaction above and beyond age (negative relationship) and living with partner status (positive relationship), which have been shown to be related to sexual satisfaction in prior research (Biss & Horne, 2005; Deeks & McCabe, 2001; Haavio-Mantila & Kontula, 1997). In addition, the relationship of sexual orientation (lesbian/queer and bisexual) was explored in relationship to sexual satisfaction.

METHOD

Participants

A total of 1257 participants completed the survey. For the purposes of the current study, participants were restricted to female participants who identified as either lesbian/queer or bisexual, identified with a faith group, and responded to the faith and sexual satisfaction measures (n = 318). The average age of participants was 36 years of age. A majority of the participants identified as Caucasian (85.8%); over 4% (4.4%) identified as Biracial/Multiracial, 3.8% as Other, 3.1% as Black/African-American, 1.3% as Asian/Asian American as well as 1.3% as Native American, and .3% as Chicano/Mexican/Mexican-American. Almost three quarters (74.8%) identified as lesbian/queer while 25.2% identified as bisexual. In terms of religious affiliation, the largest percentage of the group (49.1%) identified themselves as Other with a faith we had not listed and wrote in their faiths (including affiliations with gay affirming faith groups, Wiccans, and Pagans). The next largest group identified as Protestant (36.8%) followed by Catholic (9.1%), Jewish (4.4%), and Muslim (.6%).

Measures

Santa Clara Strength of Religious Faith Questionnaire (SCSORF; Plante & Boccaccini, 1997). The SCSORF assesses the strength of non-denominational religious faith using a 10-item questionnaire. Items are scored on a 4-point scale, ranging from 1 (strongly disagree) to 4 (strongly agree). Higher scores indicate a stronger religious faith. Plante and Boccaccini (1997) reported high internal reliability (Cronbach alpha = .95, split-half reliability r = .92) for this measure. Internal consistency was .93 for this sample.

Spiritual Wellness Inventory (SWI; Ingersoll, 1998). The SWI is a valid and reliable 55-item instrument that measures multiple dimensions of spiritual wellness: (1) conception of the absolute/divine, (2) meaning, (3) connectedness, (4) mystery, (5) spiritual freedom, (6) experience/ritual, (7) forgiveness, (8) hope, (9) knowledge/learning, and (10) present-centeredness. Due to the limited space of the survey, only subscales deemed most relevant to GLB individuals were included. The six subscales and their Cronbach alpha levels were (1) conception of the absolute/divine (α = .77), (3) connectedness (α = .65), (4) mystery (α = .41), (5) spiritual freedom (α = .70), (7) forgiveness (α = .66), and (8) hope (α = .63). Response choices are on an 8-point scale, ranging from 1 (strongly disagree) to 8 (strongly agree); higher scores represent greater levels of spiritual wellness.

Age Universal Religious Orientation Intrinsic/Extrinsic Revised Scale (I/E-R; Gorsuch & McPherson, 1989). The I/E-R scale measures intrinsic and extrinsic components of religious orientation. It is an extension of both Allport and Ross' (1967) Religious Orientation I-E scale and of Gorsuch and Venable's (1983) Age-Universal I-E Scale. It can be used with a variety of ages and includes more extensive research on the extrinsic scale. The I/E-R consists of 14 items, each with 5-point Likert-type response options. It contains three Ep (extrinsic-personal) items, three Es (extrinsic-social), and eight I (intrinsic) items. The intrinsic scale has an internal reliability of .83, while the two extrinsic subscales had low reliabilities in previous studies (Ep alpha = .57 and Es alpha = .58) with a higher combined (Es/Ep Cronbach alpha of .65) (Gorsuch & McPherson, 1989). The combined Es/Ep scale was used for this study. Higher scores indicate greater agreement with each subscale. For this study, the Cronbach alpha for the intrinsic and extrinsic scales were .77 and .63, respectively.

The Sexual Satisfaction Subscale of the Extended Satisfaction with Life Scale (ESWLS; Alfonso et al., 1996). This instrument is a 5-item, Likert-type scale that measures one's general satisfaction with sexuality as a whole. Responses ranged from 1 (strongly disagree) to 6 (strongly agree) with higher scores indicating more sexual satisfaction. Results have shown adequate internal consistency reliability (α = .96) and test-retest reliability (r = .87) as well as adequate convergent and discriminant validity for this measure. Cronbach alpha for this sample was .97.

Procedures

Participants completed an Internet study in which the stated purpose was to gain information about GLB people's spiritual and religious experiences. The Internet was used because of the often hidden nature of GLB persons and because it provides access to a larger, more diverse sample of GLB persons' experiences than other methods. The appropriateness of Internet research has been investigated and has been found to be as reliable as traditional methods of survey research, to allow people to be represented who would be unattainable if more traditional methods were used, and to improve accuracy when accessing special populations (Buchanan & Smith, 1999; Gosling et al., 2004; Kraut et al., 2004). Information about the survey was posted on GLB listserves, bulletin boards, and websites. Participants were asked to complete the survey in its entirety, had as much time as needed to complete it, and could discontinue their participation at any time. Anonymity was ensured by not collecting any identifying information, and informed consent was confirmed by submission of participant's completed responses to the survey.

RESULTS

A regression analysis was conducted to examine the potential relationship between women's faith and their reports of sexual satisfaction. A hierarchical, block-entry, regression format was used to enter variables in three stages to measure the R^2 change for each set of variables. Three blocks were entered. The first block contained three background variables of age, sexual orientation (i.e., lesbian/queer or bisexual), and living status (i.e., with partner or with someone other than a partner/alone). The next block contained three items measuring religious variables (i.e., how many times participants attended faith services, the Santa Clara Strength of Religious Faith Questionnaire, and the Intrinsic/Extrinsic Scale Revised), while the third block contained a spirituality measure (i.e., Spiritual Wellness Inventory). The dependent variable was sexual satisfaction.

Results are presented in Table 1. The model was significant ($p < .01$). The background variables accounted for 9.7% of the variance. Religion measures did not account for any significant additional variance, contributing 1.5% of the variance. However, the spirituality measure did account for a significant proportion of the variance, contributing another 2.7% of the total 14% explained variance. Three of the variables had significant influence on sexual satisfaction. These variables, in order of magnitude, were (1) living with partner or not ($\beta = -.276$), (2) intrinsic scale score ($\beta = -.234$), and (3) spiritual wellness score ($\beta = .210$). Women living with their partners reported more sexual satisfaction. There was a negative relationship between intrinsic scores and sexual satisfaction such that participants with higher scores on the intrinsic scale reported less sexual satisfaction. There was a positive relationship between spiritual wellness and sexual satisfaction, though. Women with higher levels of spiritual wellness reported greater sexual satisfaction.

Since the SWI was significant in the original regression, a second hierarchical regression was used to investigate the potential influence of its subscales on women's sexual satisfaction. Two blocks were entered for this regression. The same background variables were entered in the first block (i.e., age, sexual orientation, living status), and the six subscales of the SWI included in this study were entered into the second block (i.e., conception of the absolute/divine, connectedness, mystery, spiritual freedom, forgiveness, hope). Results are presented in Table 2. Background variables contributed 9.7% of the variance, and the SWI subscales contributed an additional 5.8% of the variance for a total of

TABLE 1. Summary of Hierarchical Regression Analysis of Faith Variables Contributing to Sexual Satisfaction in Nonheterosexual Women (n = 318)

	B	SE B	β	R	Change in R
Model 1 (Background variables only)				9.7**	
Age	−2.79E-02	.044	−.036		
Sexual Orient.	.548	1.155	.027		
Live w/partner or not	−5.607	.966	−.314*		
Model 2 (Religion variables added)				11.3	1.5
Age	−2.60E-02	.046	−.034		
Sexual Orient.	.499	1.167	.024		
Live w/partner or not	−5.580	.972	−.313**		
Church Attend.	−.176	.484	−.024		
Santa Clara	1.826E-02	.072	.017		
Model 3 (Spirituality variables added)				14**	2.7**
Age	−1.52E-02	.046	−.020		
Sexual Orient.	.411	1.147	.020		
Live w/partner or not	−4.931	.490	−.050**		
Church Attend.	−.364	.490	−.050		
Santa Clara	.124	.091	.137		
Spiritual Wellness	.200	.064	.210**		
Intrinsic	−2.827	1.191	−.234*		
Extrinsic	−.652	.839	−.045		

* $p < .02$,   ** $p < .01$

15.5% of the explained variance. Three of the variables had a significant influence on sexual satisfaction. In order of magnitude, they were (1) living with partner or not ($\beta = -.278$), (2) spiritual freedom ($\beta = .203$), and (3) connectedness ($\beta = .137$). Spiritual freedom and connectedness were the only two subscales that had a significant relationship with sexual satisfaction; both of the relationships were positive. Women who reported higher scores on the spiritual freedom subscale reported greater sexual satisfaction as did women who reported higher levels of connectedness. Again, women living with their partners reported greater sexual satisfaction.

TABLE 2. Summary of Hierarchical Regression Analysis of SWI Subscale Variables Contributing to Sexual Satisfaction in Nonheterosexual Women (n = 318)

	B	SE B	β	R	Change in R
Model 1 (Background variables only)				9.7**	
Age	−2.79E-02	.044	−.036		
Sexual Orient.	.548	1.155	.027		
Live w/partner or not	−5.607	.966	−.314*		
Model 2 (SWI subscales added)				15.5**	5.8**
Age	−5.37E-02	.044	−.070		
Sexual Orient.	.437	1.197	.021		
Live w/partner or not	−4.950	.958	−.278**		
Conception of Divine	−.303	.235	−.085		
Connectedness	.587	.291	.137*		
Mystery	−3.03E-02	.319	−.006		
Hope	−.188	.301	−.047		
Forgiveness	−1.75E-02	.268	−.004		
Spiritual Freedom	.764	.248	.203**		

* $p < .05$,   ** $p < .01$

DISCUSSION

The results of this study explained 14% of the variance in a sample of lesbian/queer and bisexual women's sexual satisfaction. Living with a partner contributed the greatest amount of variance, but spirituality also contributed to reports of sexual satisfaction, highlighting the need for researchers and therapists alike to explore a connection between faith and sex. The fact that spirituality measures significantly contributed to the variance while religion measures did not, draws attention to the importance of assessing one's spiritual connection. This incorporation may be even more salient for GLB individuals, as previous research has shown that GLB persons often value a spiritual connection more than a religious connection (e.g., Lee & Busto, 1991; Yip, 2002). The findings of this study provide suggestions for future research using qualitative methodologies to investigate the phenomenological experiences of spirituality and religion for GLB persons, and to explore the experiences of GLB persons who identify more closely with a spiritual connection than with a religious connection. These studies would shed light on the important aspects of religion and spirituality and how they relate to the experience of sexual satisfaction.

The positive relationship between spiritual wellness and sexual satisfaction was not surprising. The influence of the SWI subscales, spiritual freedom and connectedness, to sexual satisfaction can be explained by Ingersoll's (1998) description of both subscales. He stated that the spiritual freedom subscale is related to a person's capacity for play, specifically including sexual play. Based on that description, it is reasonable that a woman with a high score on that subscale would also report a higher level of sexual satisfaction. His description of what the connectedness subscale measures focused on an individual's personal connection to a spiritual being, which supports the relationship between spirituality and sexual satisfaction. It may be that a strong sense of spirituality, regardless of religious commitment or involvement, provides an individual with the capacity for spiritual connection. As research has shown, GLB persons frequently rate spiritual connection more importantly than religious affiliation; therefore, the findings support the importance of continued exploration of the role of spirituality in lesbian and bisexual women's lives, and this includes within their sexuality.

The negative relationship between intrinsic religious orientation and sexual satisfaction was a bit surprising. An explanation of these results is that spiritual wellness measures a broad, overarching connection with spirituality, whereas intrinsic and extrinsic religious orientation incorporate more religious aspects and includes specific references to church and church attendance. The negative relationship could be explained by an internalization of negative religious messages about sexuality. Historically, many religions have viewed sexuality within a narrowly defined lens, typically excluding homosexuality. Individuals who internalize such messages may experience a negative relationship between their internal religious beliefs and their sexual satisfaction. Future studies might investigate the correlation between intrinsic orientation, typically correlated positively with mental health (e.g., Richards, 1991) and sexual satisfaction for heterosexual samples.

One other result that warrants mention was the lack of influence of the age variable. The significant relationship noted in previous research of a negative relationship between age and sexual satisfaction (e.g., Deeks, & McCabe, 2001; Haavio-Mannila, & Kontula, 1997) was not evident in this study. It may be that age is less important for these women than having a partner with whom they can be sexually active and spiritually connected. Although it is assumed that women who live with their partners are sexually active, this study was based on their subjective experiences of sexual satisfaction, so little is known of their actual sexual behaviors. Sexual orientation was also not a significant predictor of sexual satisfaction, indicating that neither lesbian/queer women nor bisexual women were more likely to report greater sexual satisfaction.

While this study contributes to the field, there are several limitations. Limitations include the nature of self-report data and that only women who identified as lesbian, queer, or bisexual and were active in their faith were included. The primary limitation of self-report data is that there is no way to verify that data are accurate. However, because of the unobtrusive and anonymous nature of this project, self-report is the best means of data collection available in many cases, particularly for sensitive topics. While the findings are based on subjective experiences of these women's lives, the anonymity created by Internet collection allows people more freedom to discuss such issues more openly than they might discuss them if data was collected using a different method (Buchanan & Smith, 1999; Gosling et al., 2004; Kraut et al., 2004). The Internet also provides access to a wide population and is helpful in accessing experiences of often hidden groups, which includes lesbian, queer, and bisexual women.

At the same time that Internet data collection is beneficial, it does typically limit the sample to people of middle and upper socioeconomic statuses with access to a computer and the Internet, as was the case in this study. Thus, the study was over-represented with Caucasian participants and people with higher educational levels (e.g., Gosling et al., 2004). Although the researchers made concerted efforts to access the experiences of women of color through ethnically and racially diverse websites serving women's communities, the participation of women of color was much less than desired. LB women of color may have had less access to the Internet or may have been more reluctant to participate in a survey on sexual orientation and spirituality because of more complications and less acceptance that is believed to be experienced by some racial/ethnic groups because of the multiple intertwining prejudices of racism, ethnic discrimination, and homophobia (Greene, 1994, 1997; McCarn & Fassinger, 1996). It is expected that other findings might emerge with respect to spirituality and sexuality if a study is conducted primarily with LB women of color; therefore, these results should be taken with caution and not generalized to ethnically and racially diverse LB women's experiences. Future research should explore this area, given the conflict many ethnic minority LB women experience in relationship to their religious or sexual identities (e.g., Espin, 1997).

This study was limited in that it did not access the varied experiences of women who may not have been affiliated with a faith or who may have identified with another sexual identity. However, this study was unique in that it included a fairly large percentage of bisexual women (25.2%), who are often neglected in GLB research. The results also shed light on LB women's experiences in multiple ways. They support the prior studies showing that spirituality is important to the lives of GLB persons, and it prioritizes the role of spirituality in sexual satisfaction over the relationship of religious faith, attendance, or affiliation. Because spirituality may be even more relevant for clients, especially lesbian, queer, and bisexual clients, it is important for therapists to incorporate exploration of clients' spiritual beliefs and connections in addition to religious beliefs and connections. Although there are many other factors that may explain the overall variance in sexual satisfaction, this is one of the few studies to show the connection between spirituality and sexual satisfaction.

This study is particularly beneficial because it portrays the experiences of lesbian, queer, and bisexual women, who are often overlooked and marginalized due to their sexual orientation. Such findings showing the important connection between spirituality and sexuality may help to de-stigmatize the sexual lives of women who are romantically and sexually involved with women by clarifying that a sense of spiritual freedom and connection are important to the sexual relationship for many women, which is often a target for trivialization and objectification by popular media. Therapists may wish to explore spiritual aspects of the sexual relationship with clients and same-sex women's couples as a means of opening up discussion of a topic that is often clinically sensitive. Therapists can help expand the views of sexuality, particularly women's sexuality, by describing the spiritual aspects of sexuality in the session.

REFERENCES

Allina, A. (2001). Orgasms for sale: The role of profit and politics in addressing women's sexual satisfaction. *Women and Therapy, 24*(1-2), 211-218.

Allport, G. W., & Ross, M. W. (1967). Personal religious orientation and prejudice. *Journal of Personality and Social Psychology, 5*, 432-443.

Alfonso, V. C., Allison, D. B., Rader, D. E., & Gorman, B. S. (1996). The extended satisfaction with life scale: Development and psychometric properties. *Social Indicators Research, 38*, 275-301.

Barrett, R., & Barzan, R. (1996). Spiritual experiences of gay men and lesbians. *Counseling and Values, 41*, 4-15.

Biss, W. J. & Horne, S. G. (2005). Sexual satisfaction as more than a gendered concept: The roles of psychological well-being and sexual orientation. *Journal of Constructivist Psychology, 18*(1), 25-38.

Buchanan, T., & Smith, J. L. (1999). Using the internet for psychological research: Personality testing on the world wide web. *British Journal of Psychology, 90*, 125-144.

Byers, E. S., & Demmons, S. (1999). Sexual satisfaction and sexual self-disclosure within dating relationships. *The Journal of Sex Research, 36*(2), 180-199.

Davidson, M. G. (2000). Religion and spirituality. In Perez, R. M., DeBond, K. A., & Bieschke, K. J., *Handbook of Counseling and Psychotherapy with Lesbian, Gay and Bisexual Clients* (pp. 409-433). Washington, DC: American Psychological Association.

Deeks, A. A., & McCabe, M. P. (2001). Sexual function and menopausal women: The importance of age and partner's sexual functioning. *The Journal of Sex Research, 38*(3), 219-225.

Dunn, K. M., Croft, P. R., & Hackett, G. I. (2000). Satisfaction in the sex life of a general population sample. *Journal of Sex and Marital Therapy, 26*, 141-151.

Dupras, A. (1994). Internalized homophobia and psychosexual adjustment among gay men. *Psychological Reports, 75*, 23-28.

Ellison, G. G. (1995). Race, religious involvement and depressive symptomatology in a southeastern U.S. community. *Soc. Sci. Med., 40*, 1561-1572.

Espin, O. M. (1997). Crossing borders and boundaries: The life of narratives of immigrant Lesbians. In B. Greene (Ed.), *Ethnic and cultural diversity among lesbians and gay men* (pp. 191-215). Thousand Oaks, CA: Sage.

Gorsuch, R., & McPherson, S. E. (1989). Intrinsic/extrinsic measurement: I/E-Revised and single-item scales. *Journal for the Scientific Study of Religion, 28*, 348-354.

Gorsuch, R., & Venable, D. G. (1983). Development of an "Age Universal" I-E scale. *Journal for the Scientific Study of Religion, 22*, 181-187.

Gosling, S. D., Vazire, S., Srivastava, S. & John, O. (2004, February/March). Should we trust web-based studies? A comparative analysis of six preconceptions about internet questionnaires. *American Psychologist, 59*(2), 93-104.

Greene, B. (1994). Lesbian women of color: Triple jeopardy. In L. Comas-Díaz & B. Greene (Eds.), *Women of color: Integrating ethnic and gender identities in psychotherapy* (pp. 389-427). New York: Guilford.

Greene, B. (1997). Lesbian woman of color: Triple jeopardy. *Journal of Lesbian Studies, 1*, 109-147.

Haavio-Mannila, E., & Kontula, O. (1997). Correlates of increased sexual satisfaction. *Archives of Sexual Behavior, 26*(4), 399-420.

Howard, J. A., (1988). Gender differences in sexual attitudes: Conservatism or powerlessness? *Gender & Society, 2*(1), 103-114.

Hurlbert, D. F. (1991). The role of assertiveness in female sexuality: A comparative study between sexually assertive and sexually nonassertive women. *Journal of Sex and Marital Therapy, 17*(3), 183-190.

Hurlbert, D. F., & Apt, C. (1993). Female sexuality: A comparison study between women in homosexual and heterosexual relationships. *Journal of Sex and Marital Therapy, 19*(4), 315-327.

Ingersoll, R. E. (1998). Refining dimensions of spiritual wellness: A cross-traditional approach. *Counseling and Values, 42,* 156-165.

Koenig, H. G. (1998). *Handbook of religion and mental health.* San Diego, CA: Academic Press.

Kraut, R., Olson, J., Banaji, M., Cohen, J. & Couper, M. (2004, February/March). Psychological research online: Report of board of scientific affairs' advisory group on the conduct of research and the internet. *American Psychologist, 59*(2), 105-117.

Lease, S. H., Horne, S. G., & Noffsinger-Frazier, N. (in press). Affirming faith experiences and psychological health for Caucasian lesbian, gay, and bisexual individuals. *Journal of Counseling Psychology.*

Lease, S. & Horne, S. G. (2002). [Lesbian, gay, bisexual and transgendered (LGBT) religion and spirituality study results]. Unpublished raw data.

Lee, K. G., & Busto, R. (1991). When the spirit moves us. *OUT/LOOK, 14,* 83-85.

Levin, J. S., Markides, K. S., & Ray, L. A. (1996). Religious attendance and psychological well-being in Mexican Americans: A panel analysis of three-generations data. *The Gerontologist, 36,* 454-463.

Manley, E. D. & Horne, S. G. (2003). Religious conflict and spiritual well-being: The role of faith affiliation in the lives of gay, lesbian, and bisexual individuals. Unpublished manuscript.

McCarn, S. R., & Fassinger, R. E. (1996). Revisioning sexual minority identity formation: A new model of lesbian identity and its implications for counseling and research. *The Counseling Psychologist, 24,* 508-534.

Miller, W. M., & Thoresen, C. E. (2003). Spirituality, religion, and health: An emerging research field. *American Psychologist, 58,* 24-35.

Morrow, D. F. (2003). Cast into the wilderness: The impact of institutionalized religion on lesbians. *Journal of Lesbian Studies, 7*(4), 109-123.

Meyer, I. H., & Dean, L. (1994). Internalized homophobia, intimacy, and sexual behavior among gay and bisexual men. In B. Greene & G. M. Herek (Eds.). *Psychological perspectives on lesbian and gay issues: Vol. 1. Lesbian and gay psychology: Theory, research, and clinical applications.* (pp. 160-186). Thousand Oaks, CA: Sage.

Peplau, L. A. (2003). Human Sexuality: How do men and women differ. *Current Directions in Psychological Sciences,* 12(2), 37-40.

Peplau, L. A., & Garnets, L. D. (2000). A new paradigm for understanding women's sexuality and sexual orientation. *Journal of Social Issues, 56*(2), 329-350.

Plante, T. G., & Boccaccini, M. (1997). Reliability and validity of the Santa Clara Strength of Religious Faith Questionnaire. *Pastoral Psychology, 45,* 429-437.

Powell, L. H., Shahabi, L., & Thoresen, C. E. (2003). Religion and spirituality: Linkages to physical health. *American Psychologist, 58,* 36-52.

Richards, S. P. (1991). Religious devoutness in college students: Relations with emotional adjustment and psychological separation from parents. *Journal of Counseling Psychology, 38,* 189-196.

Rose, E. M., Westefeld, J. S., & Ansely, T. N. (2001). Spiritual issues in counseling: Clients' beliefs and preferences. *Journal of Counseling Psychology, 48*(1), 61-71.

Rose, S. (1996). Lesbian and gay love scripts. In E. D. Rothblum & L. A. Bond (Eds.). *Preventing heterosexism and homophobia* (pp. 151-173). Thousand Oaks, CA: Sage.

Ross, C. E. (1990). Religion and psychological distress. *Journal for the Scientific Study of Religion, 29*, 236-245.

Schuck, K. D. & Liddle, B. J. (2001). Religious conflicts experienced by lesbian, gay, and bisexual individuals. *Journal of Gay and Lesbian Psychotherapy, 5*(2), 63-81.

Smith, B. L. & Horne, S. G. (in press). Gay, lesbian, bisexual and transgendered (GLBT) experiences with earth-spirited faiths. *Journal of Homosexuality.*

Sprecher, S. (2002). Sexual satisfaction in premarital relationships: Associations with satisfaction, love, commitment, and stability. *The Journal of Sex Research, 39*(3), 190-196.

Sue, D. W., Bingham, R. P., Porche-Burke, L., & Vasquez, M. (1999). The diversification of psychology: A multicultural revolution. *American Psychologist, 54*(12), 1061-1069.

Tiefer, L. (2001). Arriving at a "New View" of women's sexual problems: Background, theory, and activism. *Women & Therapy, 24*, 63-98.

Ventis, W. L. (1995). The relationships between religion and mental health. *Journal of Social Issues, 51*, 33-48.

Williamson, I. R. (2000). Internalized homophobia and health issues affecting lesbians and gay men. *Health Education Research, 15*(1), 97-107.

Worthington, E. L., Karusu, T. A., McCullough, M. E., & Sandage, S. J. (1996). Empirical research on religion and psychotherapeutic processes and outcomes: A 10-year review and research prospectus. *Psychological Bulletin, 119*, 448-487.

Yip, A. K. T. (2002). The persistence of faith among nonheterosexual christians: Evidence for the neosecularization thesis of religious transformation. *Journal for the Scientific Study of Religion, 41*(2), 199-212.

Young, M., Denny, G., Young, T., & Luquis, R. (2000). Sexual satisfaction among married women. *American Journal of Health Studies, 16*(2), 73-84.

Is It Possible
for Christian Women to Be Sexual?

Amy Mahoney

SUMMARY. A qualitative semi-structured interview was used to explore the interaction between Christian women's sexuality and spirituality and the impact of sex-negative messages on sexual and spiritual development of 10 Caucasian, middle-aged Christian women. A salient feature of this negative interaction was the women's attempts to reduce the dissonance between their sexuality and spirituality, which reflected a developmental process. Results are discussed in terms of the difficulty Christian women face in being able to integrate their sexuality and spirituality. The study revealed that integration is not an end but an ongoing process. Clinical implications and recommendations for future research are offered.

Amy Mahoney is employed at a non-profit agency in San Diego, CA.

But the beginning of things, of a world, especially,
Is necessarily vague, tangled, chaotic, and exceedingly disturbing.
How few of us ever emerge from such a beginning!
How many souls perish in its tumult! (Kate Chopin, 1899)

INTRODUCTION

Sister Ann sat before her priest/confessor in great emotional turmoil as she related to him the conflict she was enduring. The young Sister was experiencing troubling thoughts and feelings of a sexual nature. She had already taken a perpetual vow of celibacy, and weren't such thoughts and feelings a sign that she was not being true to her vow? Did this mean her vocation was in jeopardy? The conflict for Sister Ann was between two mutually exclusive identities–spirituality and sexuality. She had been taught that as a Christian woman, she should strive for perfection and imitation of the Virgin Mary. She was also taught that sex was sinful and sexual thoughts and feelings were to be overcome by a strong and pure spiritual devotion for God alone. Moreover, the nature of her sexual feelings was most troubling because she was feeling attracted to another one of the Sisters. This surely was sinful and meant that she was not only in a crisis of vocation, but her very soul was at stake because of the perversion of her desires.

What Sister Ann discovered with the help of a feminist psychologist during several years of therapy after leaving her convent is that her vow to be celibate had been based on an assumed heterosexual identity, which meant nothing to her. Without conscious awareness, Sister Ann embraced an asexual identity because she could not accept a homosexual identity and she was not attracted to men. Her promise to be celibate for the love of God was not a sacrifice for her because she had rejected sexuality altogether, though she did not realize it, and certainly at the time she made her perpetual vows she did not have the benefit of this awareness. Sister Ann could not be heterosexual or homosexual so her default choice was asexual.

The story of Sister Ann is not uncommon among women who have been members of religious communities. It is not uncommon to hear women in general describe the task of clarifying and integrating their sexual and spiritual identity as challenging, risky, and scary.

In 1899, Kate Chopin wrote a story titled *The Awakening*. When it was published, it created a scandal because of its open treatment of the topic of a woman's sensuality and suicide. The story is about a married woman who develops a romantic interest in another man. In the end, the woman commits suicide. *The Awakening* has been reclaimed as a feminist classic and new framings of the story's themes and ending have been suggested (Christ, 1980).

Sister Ann first read this story in 1980 when she was a nun in a cloistered monastery. You may have guessed by now that I am Sister Ann. Since that time, I have returned to *The Awakening* again and again because the courageous struggle of the protagonist, Edna Pontellier, always inspired me at challenging and difficult times in my life, especially when I was facing a crisis of vocation and considering leaving my monastery. The essence of Chopin's protagonist is Edna's quest for wholeness—for integration of sexual and creative passion as a woman. There is a specific moment in Edna's awakening, as she walks by the sea, the medium of her awakening that has always been very poignant to me. As Christ (1980) notes, it is at this moment of nearness to the power of the sea that Edna can feel the boundless potential of her soul and begins to question her life.

My interest in the effects of the dichotomization of sexuality and spirituality in women's lives emerged from the ashes of my personal awakening to the damaging effects of Western Christian socialization in my own life. My awakening led me to believe that the integration of sexuality and spirituality is necessary precisely because people see them as separate for the most part. Many Christian women have grown up with the message that they can be spiritual, but not sexual or they can be sexual, but not spiritual. They cannot be both simultaneously. They must give up one in order to be the other. They can be like the Madonna (and this is preferred) or if they express sexual pleasure and freedom, they will likely be considered "loose" women. A Christian woman's destiny, upon which her eternity depends, is to become a man's wife, bear his children, and take care of everyone but herself. Edna could not do it, and I wonder how many other women have followed Edna into the sea, literally and figuratively, because they could not do it either.

I believe the principles of feminist psychotherapy as articulated by Kaschak (1992) are particularly well suited for developing an integrated approach to women's sexuality and spirituality. Such an approach to therapy provides a radical understanding of the damaging effects of the patriarchal culture in which we live. Kaschak states that feminist psychotherapies and epistemologies "are both oriented toward exposing masculinist meanings and their damaging effects in general and in particular, and toward developing alternative meanings and choices based upon the actual lived experience of girls and women" (Kaschak, 1992, p. 210).

The practice of feminist therapy is based on multicultural feminist scholarship and methodologies that support multiple ways of knowing. "It is a practice informed by ways of seeing, knowing, feeling, and understanding rooted in the refusal of feminism to accept the dominant culture as a healthy or worthwhile model for human behavior" (Brown, 1994, p. 49). A feminist therapy perspective can facilitate reparative reconnections for women's psycho/sexual/spiritual growth and development "by viewing women's experience and ways of knowing positively and centrally" (Ballou, 1990). Dualistic, negative thinking that has compartmentalized women's sexuality and spirituality in terms of Madonna or whore must be replaced with positive alternatives arising from women's own experience and definitions of their sexuality and spirituality. Mary Hunt, cofounder and codirector of the Women's Alliance for Theology, Ethics, and Ritual (WATER), would frame such alternatives in terms of social and sexual justice for women (Hunt, 2001). Alternatives to the traditional andocentric views of sexuality must be developed that offer women the possibility of discovering and integrating the spiritual dimensions of sexuality. Such alternatives can help to develop positive understandings of sexuality that will empower women to become fully, passionately alive to their sexuality and provide a sense of empowerment and freedom rather than fear of abuse and exploitation.

"Carl Jung once remarked that when people brought sexual questions to him they invariably turned out to be religious questions, and when they brought religious questions to him they always turned out to be sexual ones." (Nelson, 1978, p. 14). Jung was not alone in concluding that issues related to a person's concerns about sexuality could turn out to be spiritual questions and vis-à-vis. Helminiak (1987) argues, "when spirituality is thought to encompass the integration of all aspects of the person and the resultant actualization of one's fullest potential, the role of sexuality in one's spiritual development becomes obvious and pressing" (Helminiak, 1989, p. 201).

More recently, sex researcher and marriage and family therapist Gina Ogden (1997) conducted a national survey specifically to explore the connection between sexuality and spirituality. All together, she received 3,810 completed surveys along with 1,465 narrative responses from women and men who reported they were eager to explore their experiences of the relationship between sexuality and spirituality.

I recently conducted a study to explore the ways women socialized in Western Christian Culture experience challenges and conflict in the process of integrating their sexuality and spirituality.[1] The study recruited participants through fliers passed out to local Christian women's groups, psychologists and other licensed therapists, and local colleges and universities. Data collection consisted of two parts, both taking place on the same day. In the first part, the participants were asked to complete a demographic questionnaire and an introductory warm-up activity pertaining to their sexuality and spirituality. This activity was intended to facilitate participants' memory of past thoughts and feelings about their sexuality and spirituality prior to the start of the interview. The second part consisted of an audiotape, semi-structured interview consisting of 10 questions.

Ten women, all of them Caucasian, participated in this study and each was given a pseudonym to protect confidentiality. Seven of the women were raised Roman Catholic and three were raised in other Christian denominations, namely Methodist, Congregational, and Baptist. At the time of their interviews, only three of the seven women who indicated they were raised Catholic said they still considered themselves Roman Catholic. The other three women said their current religious affiliations were Metaphysical, Evangelical, or none. Four of the women identified their sexual orientation as bi-sexual, three as heterosexual, and three as lesbian. Nine of the women were married at least once, four were married more than once, and one woman was married 5 times.

INDIVIDUAL DESCRIPTIONS
OF THE WOMEN INTERVIEWED

Nan is 63 years old, and works as an administrator for a large corporation. She said, "Today I consider myself 'bisexual.'" She has been in a committed relationship with her female partner for 10 years. She was raised Roman Catholic, but left the Church after 28 years and said, "My spirituality follows a metaphysical path at this point in my life." *Mary* is 57 years old, and is employed as a healthcare administrator. She was raised Roman Catholic, but no longer considers herself Catholic and has no formal religious affiliation at this time in her life. She was married for 12 years, divorced, and has been in a committed relationship with her female partner for 13 years. *Laura* is 55 years old, retired, and has been married to her husband for 34 years. She was raised Methodist, but said, "Once I got married my husband directed the course of our lives and he didn't go to Church so I stopped going and sort of drifted away all together." *Louise* is 54 years old, works as a researcher at a local University, and has been married to her 5th husband for the past 17 years.

She was raised Roman Catholic, but when she left home at 18, she left the Catholic Church. At age 33, she rededicated herself to God and began attending a non-denominational Christian Church. *Jinny* is 62 years old, and employed as a health educator. She was raised Roman Catholic and has remained in the Catholic Church throughout her life. She divorced after 24 years of marriage and has been in a committed relationship with her female partner for 10 years. *Melissa* is 46 years old, works in the human services field, and was married and divorced twice. She grew up Roman Catholic, but fell away from the Church in college when "I started drinking and having sex." She found God and spirituality again after "I became sober through Alcoholic Anonymous." *Jeane* is 72 years old, retired, and was raised in "A very strict Catholic household by my grandparents." She graduated from high school in 1949 and married the same year. She divorced after 26 years of marriage. She has been living in a committed relationship with her female partner for 24 years. *Anna* is 49 years old, and is employed in the healthcare field. She was raised in the Congregational Church and was married and divorced twice. *Anna's* second marriage ended when "I discovered I was attracted to women and I had an affair with a woman." At age 40, she converted to Catholicism. *Anna* considers herself "bisexual" and has been in a committed relationship with her female partner for six years. *Xena* is 48 years old, single, and is employed by the government. She is lesbian and has been dating a woman for about 12 months. She grew up in a Baptist/Christian household in which religion was "a big part of my family experience." At age 19, *Xena* said "goodbye to patriarchal religion" and embraced goddess spirituality. *Bernadette* is 52 years old, and employed as an educator. She grew up in a Catholic family and remains in the Catholic Church. *Bernadette's* first marriage lasted seven years. She stated, "I got married because I had sex with by boyfriend and I believed that if I had sex I had to get married." The marriage was annulled (officially dissolved by the Catholic Church, enabling her to marry again in the Catholic Church). Her second marriage lasted 20 years and also ended in divorce. *Bernadette* described herself as "bisexual" and has been in a committed relationship with her female partner for the past six years.

The women in this study were told that the focus of the study was to explore their experience of how "they integrated their sexuality and spirituality." The study focused on (1) how their Christian beliefs influenced the development of their sexuality and spirituality, and (2) an exploration of their experience of how they have integrated their sexuality and spirituality.

RESULTS

My study began with the intent to recruit and interview Christian women who indicated by self-report that they had experienced conflict between their sexuality and spirituality, had resolved the conflict, and had been able to "integrate" their sexuality and spirituality. Despite the fact that during the phone screening all the women stated that they had resolved the conflict between their sexuality and spirituality and felt they were able to integrate their sexuality and spirituality, what quickly surfaced in the women's interviews was the persistence of conflict and contradiction.

I had expected that the women interviewed would be able to talk about the connection between their sexuality and spirituality to varying degrees since all the women were informed in the phone screening that the focus of the study was on how they integrated their sexuality and spirituality. Three of the women (*Melissa, Laura, and Bernadette*) said in the phone screening that they did not experience conflict. Nevertheless, during their interviews, all of the women expressed conflict between their sexuality and spirituality at some point in their lives. This finding suggests that even for women who have or believe they have been able to integrate their sexuality and spirituality, the fact is that they encountered obstacles of religious and secular social control with which they had to struggle before they could integrate their sexuality and spirituality. Moreover, the fact that they did not initially acknowledge the conflict also suggests that these women tolerated and overcame experiences that they did not initially describe or recognize as conflictual.

It became clear that the issue of conflict between sexuality and spirituality first began for these women in early adolescence. What brought the internal conflict into focus was awareness that their sexual behavior was inconsistent with their Christian religious traditions. The women articulated the conflict between their sexuality and spirituality, but were less able to describe how they integrated their sexuality and spirituality. They found it hard to articulate those moments in which they experienced "feeling" and "being" integrated. *Jinny* commented, "it's really hard to describe, it's a warm feeling, like floating close to heaven." *Xena* reflected, "it's a feeling, it's just a feeling, it's an essence." At the time of their interview, with the exception of *Bernadette*, most of the women felt that their sexuality and spirituality were integrated in their lives today and that both these domains operate as a function of who they perceive themselves to be. They believe they have been able to make this integration as a result of a journey of conflict resolution, and in this respect, they have been able to integrate their sexuality and spirituality.

It was an assumption of this study that women socialized in Western Christian culture would experience conflict between their sexuality and spirituality. This conflict is the legacy of dualistic thinking that stated that the body is inferior, the mind/or soul is superior, and that sex and women are dangerous. Core values, beliefs, and attitudes about sexuality and spirituality are deeply embedded in the symbols and rituals of Western Christian tradition. Historically, the idea of an inferior human body and negative attitudes and beliefs about sexuality did not originate with Christianity, but were already present in Greek and Roman cultures. They would later be fully embraced by Christianity. Modern Christian sexual morality continues to feel the anthropological echo of such dualism as is evidenced by these women's testimonies. Combining sexuality and spirituality was not a birthright, but rather a battle fought and won by most of the women interviewed, but still being fought by others.

DISSONANCE: THE CONFLICTUAL RELATIONSHIP BETWEEN SEXUALITY AND SPIRITUALITY

The women described their conflict between sexuality and Christian teachings in a variety of ways as illustrated by some of their statements: "you do not have full blown sex until you are married or that's a sin," "I tried to put the spiritual thing aside, and just turn a switch in my head that would make me into a sexual being," and "my church taught that the woman was submissive to the man and sex was a woman's duty no matter what." As adolescents, the women said they were curious about sex and also felt peer pressure to become sexually active. This created conflict within their peer groups and put them at odds with the authority of their Christian tradition. Dissonance theory (Festinger, 1957) postulates that pairs of cognitions can be relevant or irrelevant to one another. Relevant cognitions are either consonant, meaning one follows the other, or dissonant, meaning they are the opposite. In the case of the women interviewed, the opposition between Christian messages of virginity and abstinence and their adolescent sexual curiosity and exploration caused dissonance. The existence of the dissonance created psychological discomfort, which led participants to seek different ways of reducing the conflict. *Xena* said she used "mind games," and *Nan, Melissa, Jinny, Jeane, and Bernadette* used defenses such as denial and repression. *Anna* said she used the pill. Moreover, *Xena, Melissa, and Louise* simply were not sufficiently restrained by church proscriptions and their attitudes about sex were more consonant with their peer group expectations to be sexually active. In adolescence, most of the women interviewed tolerated the tension between Christian teachings and their decisions to be sexually active in spite of the Church teachings against sex before marriage. The deeper moral questions and the need to be consistent in their beliefs and behaviors would emerge in their young adult years when most of them were married.

The women stated during their interviews that they did not start out with the awareness that there was a separation between their sexuality and spirituality. The messages about "no sex before marriage" and, "sex only with one's husband" came through the teaching authority of their religions traditions and their parents. As adolescents, they were paying more attention to not getting pregnant than to these messages. However, they were not immune to the psychological "tug-of-war" between what the voice of authority was saying and what they were actually doing. *Melissa* said,

> Well, the first time was in high school with this boyfriend who I was totally in love with and it was like if you love somebody this is what you do. Then in college, it was more like well if you want a second date you have sex, and then I stopped thinking about my religion. I mean I think I mostly had the idea that I was now evil and was going to hell anyway.

Most of the interviewees stated that trying to resolve the conflict between their sexuality and spirituality was not an intentional or even conscious process, but rather one of "discovery" as a result of conflict. As adolescents, when confronted with the conflict between religious or parental authority versus peer pressure and the need to conform, they opted for sexuality. Through the discovery and exploration of the psycho/sexual/spiritual source of the conflict, the women began a process of growth toward integration that involved looking at their lives retrospectively and evaluating their lives with a view to the redevelopment of their sexual, moral, and spiritual identities.

Nan shared an experience of a sexual encounter with a woman early on in her marriage. The "passionate nature" of the sexual experience was something she had never experienced with her husband. Twenty-eight years later, after her divorce, *Nan* said she began to explore sexual relationships with women.

At this point in my life I firmly believe that sexuality is certainly
something God created as part of who we are as human beings. I
don't feel any guilt about it in my relationship. I am monogamous
with my partner and it's a pleasurable thing and I think God intended it to be pleasurable.

The spiritual aspects of this discovery process arose in the women's lives
after they had experienced problems in their marriages. *Bernadette* said,

My second marriage was low on intimacy. I tried to put the spiritual thing aside and just turn a switch in my head that would make
me into a sexual being. I was definitely leaving the spiritual part of
me behind.

For *Nan*, prolonged turmoil in her marriage led her to seek support in
a deeper spiritual path. She stated,

The good part of it is I'm not sure if I had not been that unhappy in
my marriage if my spirituality would have grown as much as it did.
I think through that unhappiness I grew even closer in my spiritual
walk. I had what is known as a born again experience, gave my life
to God, which opened all kinds of new doors for my spiritual walk
in life. When I think back it's probably the main thing that gave me
the courage to finally break from the marriage.

CHURCH AS PARENT

Many of the women in this study talked about how chaotic their families of origin were and how "unsafe" they felt in them. In contrast, the
Church appeared as a well-organized and reliable "family" where authority lines were clearly defined and stable. It was not surprising that
the women interviewed made a connection between their family of origin
and their Christian Church since both were so closely associated when
they were growing up. The study showed a link between high family
dysfunction, high Church authority, and low sexual and spiritual satisfaction. The women whose families of origin had problems related to alcohol addiction, sexual abuse, and other forms of violence and abuse
seemed to rely more on the Church to give them the structure and stability they did not have in their families. The more dysfunctional the family, the more they sought safety and comfort in the routines and predictable

rituals of their Church. Later, after they were married, the same structure that comforted them in their childhood seemed to oppress them in adulthood. This fact was demonstrated by several women (*Nan, Melissa, Jinny, Bernadette, Jeane, and Mary*) who remained in unhappy marriages because their Church said it was their duty and divorce separated them from full participation in the life of the Church. The women who relied heavily on the Church to provide safety and security had a harder time developing their personal conscience and their moral judgments, thoughts, and behaviors regarding sexuality and spirituality. *Mary* captured this dilemma in the following statement,

> I was taught that you have spirituality through religion and if you want to be a spiritual person you got that through the church, you got one (spirituality) through the other (the church), there wasn't any other way. I didn't know how to think so I accepted that. It's like you don't know what you don't know until you know you don't know it.

One important example of the parental overtones in their experience and understanding of the Church mixed in with their experience of sexual/spiritual development arises from the figure of "father" in the Church and in the family. All the women reported their understanding of their Christian God to be "like a father, old, white hair, white beard, scary." The women in this study experienced an array of negative experiences related to either biological or stepfathers. Fathers were often contradictory figures who did not responsibly fulfill their roles as "head of the family." The fact that fathers were not more involved in the spiritual life of the family was noticed and commented on by most of the women interviewed. They wanted their fathers involved and it confused them that they did not participate in something that was ostensibly stated as an important family value. Their unreliable and sometimes abusive fathers contributed to a confused image of a God/Father that had consequences for their spiritual development.

SILENCE ABOUT SEX AND ITS ROLE
IN THE DEVELOPMENT OF THE CONFLICT

Nine of the 10 women interviewed said they received no sex education and the topic was never discussed in their homes or with their parents. These women felt that the silence regarding sexual behavior created naiveté, ambivalence, and vulnerability as they entered the arena of adolescence and faced the daunting task of upholding Christian moral values against adolescent sexual exploration. This left them ill prepared for the sexual challenges of adolescence and for the sexual and relational experiences of marriage. *Mary* commented, "I didn't have a clear sense of what sex was because nobody explained it to me." For many of the women, the extent of their sex education was a video about menstruation shown at their schools. Their mothers either did not discuss menstruation at all or simply helped them with the "mechanics" of how to use pads and belts. There was never any discussion about pregnancy or sexuality related to the start of menstruation. Again, *Mary* illustrated the point with her question, "why bleed if it doesn't mean anything?" *Jeane* said her mother told her menstruation meant she was a woman, but she did not understand what that meant nor did her mother elaborate. Against a void of information about sexuality, these women all began adolescence with the religious imperative not to engage in sexual behavior versus the social imperative of adolescent development and sexual exploration. As adolescents, they were more concerned about not getting pregnant than about the religious and moral consequences of their sexual activity. By adulthood, 8 out of the 10 women were struggling with difficult marriages.

Six of the 10 women said that sex with their husbands was not desirable or pleasurable and they were not able to successfully communicate these feelings to their husbands. *Bernadette* said she tried to talk about this with her husband, but he repeatedly refused to listen. *Mary* said her husband could not accept that she wanted to initiate sexual contact and he never allowed her to do so. *Nan's* husband was very conservative and he always decided when they had sex and their "love making" was always the same, "at night, before bed, in the dark, with him on top." *Melissa's* husband was a devout Mormon and believed she should be submissive to him. *Jinny* said it wasn't until she and her husband were in marriage counseling that she was able to tell him she did not have orgasms. *Jeane* said she was rarely orgasmic in her 26-year marriage and often "faked it." It is interesting to note that during adolescence and early adulthood, many of the women said they felt they could "control" the sexual behavior of the boys and men in their lives by telling them they would not do certain things such as vaginal or anal intercourse or oral sex. Once married, however, they lost their sexual agency, which came under the authority of their husbands. They were not able to make their voices heard or understood in the private sphere of their sexual relations with their husbands. They felt their sexual desires and needs did not have the priority or authority of their husbands' who had the power to define the terms of their sexual relationship. *Mary* reported she became angry and resentful.

> This caused a certain amount of anger and resentment and upset in our marriage. Other women could get their husbands to have sex with them and I couldn't get my husband to have sex with me so there must be something wrong with me. Of course this didn't mean we were not having sex, it just was on his terms, and it was definitely in the dark and not in the middle of the day.

Jinny commented,

> No, I never said anything about not having orgasms or not liking our sexual intimacy until we went to a marriage encounter. Then it finally came out how I felt. Then one night we were in the middle of having sex, and he starts praying that I have an orgasm. Talk about a turnoff.

Silence about sex resonated in other ways in which the women expressed that their thoughts, feelings, and voices were not affirmed. *Laura* was a prime example of a voice silenced and the meaning of her sexual experiences reinterpreted by men; two of the men were priests and the other, her husband. *Bernadette's* husband silenced her through the use of emotionally abusive statements that characterized her as a "frigid, pathetic woman" when she objected to certain sexual practices.

Silence about sex has been a destructive element in the evolution of Western Christianity. This silence and a lack of awareness about how Western Christianity has linked sex and sin and developed a sex-negative morality has perpetuated feelings of guilt and shame about human sexuality for both women and men. Silence on the part of Christian leaders about human sexuality has created a contradiction between what is taught by Christian traditions and what is practiced in the lives of many Christian women. The threads of silence were woven into these women's consciousness within their Christian families of origin. Long after they left their families of origin and married, the threads of a sex-negative Christian morality continued to impact their sexual thoughts, feelings, and behavior.

SEXUAL MOLESTATION

The most serious issue reported by the women interviewed regarding silence about sex was childhood sexual molestation, which was voluntarily reported by three of the 10 women in this study. Two other women shared enough information to suggest that they may have also been sexually abused. It is well documented in the literature that childhood sexual abuse profoundly disrupts development of normal relationships. Repeated trauma in childhood forms and deforms the personality (Herman, 1992). Herman points out that the pathological environment of childhood abuse causes the development of extraordinary coping mechanisms, some creative and some destructive. Abused children hope that growing up will enable them to escape and find freedom. Instead, what the survivor takes into adolescence and adult life are fundamental problems with basic trust, autonomy, intimacy, major impairments in self-care, and a diminished capacity to form stable relationships. *Louise*, who was married and divorced four times by the age of thirty-three, was the only participant willing to discuss the impact of her abuse experience. She reported that her paternal grandfather abused her from the time she was 6 until she was 10. She also believed that both her parents knew about the abuse "on some level." To this day, *Louise* said there is a shroud of silence about her grandfather even though he is now deceased. As an adult, *Louise* said she used sex as "a weapon" and she "seduced" her way through life. She stated there were certain aspects of sexual behavior that were very distorted and unpleasant for her.

> It (the abuse) made me not want to do things. So, I asked God to heal me of that and to take away any negative associations and to let me really enjoy my husband and have every part of him be something that is appealing to me. And that prayer has been answered. For me it was quite a leap because I had to go from some very negative associations.

Louise is fortunate in that she has been able to move forward and to regain a sense of trust in her sexual relationship with her husband. She has the capacity to take pleasure in life and to engage in satisfying and fulfilling sexual intimacy with her husband. She left no doubt that she attributed her well-being to her faith in God's power to heal and restore her damaged sexuality.

SEXUAL MINORITY ORIENTATION

Seven of the 10 participants reported a sexual minority orientation. Three women reported a lesbian sexual orientation and four women reported a bisexual orientation. While sexual orientation was not a focus of the study, and the women were not asked specifically about sexual orientation, it did emerge during their interviews. It is worth speculating about the extent to which issues of sexual orientation factor into the experience of how Christian women resolve the conflict between their sexuality and spirituality.

Flyers advertising the study invited the participation of women who were interested in exploring sexuality and spirituality. It is possible that women for whom sexual orientation was a salient feature of their identity consolidation were drawn to the study. It is also possible that the conflict between sexuality and spirituality has been a life-long challenge for sexual minority Christian women. Such women may be more likely to seek opportunities to further explore their experience. The fact that heterosexual orientation, which is considered the norm in Western culture, is not thought of as "acquired" or socially constructed, but rather as "natural." For heterosexual women, no such self-consciousness exists regarding their sexual orientation. Unless a woman deviates from the "natural" path, she is less likely to face the challenge that confronts those struggling to sort out the complexities of an alternative sexual orientation. The seven women who reported sexual minority orientation are all currently living in committed relationships with women. Issues of sexual orientation combined with Christian identity development may have sensitized and prompted these women to explore the challenges of disentangling the multiple facets of sexuality and the challenges one is faced with by Western Christian religious traditions.

CLINICAL IMPLICATIONS

There was an inverse relationship between the amount of importance given to the authority of the Christian Churches in the women's lives and the level of sexual/spiritual satisfaction they were able to experience at different points in their lives. A useful standpoint for clinicians throughout the work of therapy is helping women realize that sexual and spiritual growth is a developmental process that can be understood as interactive throughout the life span. I agree with Timmerman (1992) that there is a spiritual significance to human sexuality and a sexual significance to

spirituality in that both sexuality and spirituality can address the transcendent nature of human experience. Assessing the impact of how
these two domains function in negative and positive ways is an important clinical consideration.

The Journal of American Medicine (1999) reported that 32% of the
women interviewed in their National Health and Social Life Survey reported a lack of interest in sex, 26% said they regularly did not have orgasms, and 23% stated sex was not pleasurable. The negative impact of
religion on women's sexual development may be a factor in these figures.

The evidence provided by the literature on women's sex surveys (Davis,
1929; Hite, 1976; Laumann et al., 1999; Mosher, 1892) supports the fact
that many women are not happy with their sex lives. Yet, as recently as
2002, the scientific communities agree that not much is known about
women's sexuality. The traditional focus of sex research on the more
easily measured aspects of physical arousal, and the focus of medicine
on physiological functioning and pharmaceutical solutions has missed
the deeper emotional, psychological, spiritual, and relational aspects such
as love, tenderness, safety, and trust which women report as equally
important, and sometimes more important, than the genital/physical aspect of sex. These elements, I contend, make up the spiritual dimension
of sexuality that is extremely important to a woman's sexual satisfaction. In the exploration of the affective, relational aspects of sexuality,
women's spirituality emerges as a salient factor in understanding their
experience.

It is my contention that Western Christian women presenting for treatment in clinical settings with problems of sexual dysfunction and desire
may be experiencing conflict about sexual expectations and behaviors
which are rooted in religious values that are hard to access or approach
in a clinical setting. In doing psychotherapy with women raised in Western
Christian religious traditions, psychotherapist should be aware of this
possibility. Religious background and spirituality are often considered
in clinical assessment from the standpoint of a helpful network of social
support under difficult circumstances. I believe it may also be an area of
assessment that can hold clues to hidden problems related to sexuality
and sexual functioning for Christian women.

When conflict emerges between a woman's stated formal religious
beliefs and her articulation of her lived experience this conflict may be
obvious to the therapist but not to the client. Therapists will need to as-
sess the relevance of exploring the conflicting beliefs in light of the agreed
upon treatment goals. There may be cases in which integration of these
contradictions may not be possible, as demonstrated by the case of

Bernadette. *Bernadette* was not able to explore the relevance of the formal religious and doctrinal sex education she received in childhood in order to adjust or accommodate her lived experience as an adult in the context of a sexual/spiritual relationship with her female partner. In such a case, it will be important for the therapist to hold the tension with the client rather than eliminate the conflict. Exploration of such tension can facilitate further discovery of the core elements of the intrapsychic contradictions.

CONCLUSION

This study suggests that the challenge of integrating sexuality and spirituality for Western Christian women is a complex process involving sexual and spiritual identities, which may, at different times throughout their lives, be in opposition. Moreover, sexual satisfaction could be compromised by unexamined Christian religious values, which are not consciously understood as influencing psycho/sexual/spiritual behavior. Exploration of these values may hold clues to unlocking unconscious influences over Christian women's sexual and spiritual satisfaction.

One of my goals was to further the dialogue about women's sexuality and the importance of understanding the role of spirituality in the ongoing enlightenment about the complexities of human sexuality. It is my belief that sexuality and spirituality have more in common than in opposition. I also believe that Christian denominations hold in common that human life is sacred, that humans are made in the image of God, and that there is an eternal destiny for everyone. Sexuality is part of our God-given common human experience that I believe is meant to be shared in the "presence of God."

Sexuality has been imprinted in our cultural and social context in terms of the physicality of sex. It is my hope that this study will contribute to raising the volume of theological and scientific dialogue on how women as well as men can learn to integrate sexuality and spirituality.

ACKNOWLEDGMENTS

1. The author wants to thank Drs. Oliva Espín, Peter Wayson, and Katherine DiFrancesca for their contributions to her doctoral dissertation upon which this article is based.

REFERENCES

Ballou, M. (1990). Approaching a feminist-principled paradigm in the construction of personality theory. In L. S. Brown & M. P. P. Root (Eds.), *Diversity and complexity in feminist therapy* (pp. 23-40). New York: Haworth.

Brown, L. S. (1994). *Subversive Dialogues: Theory in Feminist Therapy*. New York: BasicBooks.

Chopin, K. (1899). *The Awakening*. Chicago: Herbert S. Stone and Company.

Christ, C. P. (1997). *Rebirth of the Goddess: Finding Meaning in Feminist Spirituality*. New York: Addison-Wesley Publishing Company, Inc.

Christ, C. P. (1980). *Diving Deep and Surfacing: Women Writers on Spiritual Quest*. Boston: Beacon Press.

Davis, K. B. (1929). *Facets in the Sex Life of Twenty-Two Hundred Women*. New York: Harper & Brothers Publishers.

Festinger, L. (1957). A Theory of Cognitive Dissonance. California: Stanford University Press.

Helminiak, D. A. (1989). Self-Esteem, Sexual Self-Acceptance, and Spirituality. *Journal of Sex Education & Therapy, 15* (No. 3), 200-210.

Herman, J. L. (1992). Trauma and Recovery. New York: BasicBooks.

Hite, S. (1976). *The Hite Report: A nationwide study of female sexuality*. New York: Macmillan.

Hunt, M. E. (2001). Just Good Sex: Feminist Catholicism and Human Rights. In P.B. Jung, M. E. Hunt, & R. Balakrishnan (Eds.). *Good Sex: Feminist Perspectives from the World's Religions* (pp. 158-173). New Jersey: Rutgers University Press.

Kaschak, E. (1992). Engendered Lives: A New Psychology of Women's Experience. New York: BasicBooks.

Laumann, E . O., Paik, A., & Rosen, R. (1999). Sexual Dysfunction in the United States: Prevalence and Predictors. *The Journal of Sex Research,* 10:281, 537-544.

Mosher, Clelia Duel (1892). *Statistical study of the marriages of forth-seven women*. Microfilm. Redwood City, California: Mark Larwood, 1975 I reel. Originals at Stanford University Archives.

Nelson, J. B. (1978). *Embodiment: An Aapproach to Sexuality and Christian Theology*. Minneapolis: Augsburg Publishing House.

Ogden, G. (1997). *Women, Sex, and the Search for God.*Paper presented at the American Psychological Association, Chicago, Illinois, Palmer House, Hilton, Session 3036.

Timmerman, J. J. (1992). *Sexuality and Spiritual Growth*. New York: Crossroad Publishing Company.

It's Not Just a Headache, Dear: Why Some Women Say No to Connecting Sex and Spirit

Gina Ogden

SUMMARY. Why do women say no to connecting sex and spirit, even though this connection is arguably self-affirming, loving, satisfying, and potentially life transforming? This paper looks for answers in the context of four cultural dynamics in which women's resistance is rooted: selective education, religious belief systems, norms about pleasure, and mind-body separation. Further, it discusses how therapists can challenge these dynamics and find teachable moments to support women's choices for whole-person sex-spirit integration. Information is based on the author's practice of sex therapy since the mid 1970s and on the nationwide survey she conducted in 1997-8, the first to investigate integrating sexuality and spirituality.

Gina Ogden is a licensed marriage and family therapist, sex therapy diplomate, and researcher at Cambridge, MA.

INTRODUCTION

We can probably all cite dozens of reasons why women say no to sex that hurts and objectifies them. But why do some women say no to connecting sex and spirit, which is arguably self-affirming, satisfying, and potentially life-transforming (Brock, 1988; Heyward, 1989; Bonheim, 1997; Beattie-Jung, Hunt, & Balakrishnan, 2001; Wade, 2004)? When women connect sex and spirit, they speak of a synergy of physical sensation with intangible experiences such as love, passion, compassion, altruism, empathy, reverence, and sometimes grace. They speak of sexual energy opening "windows to the universe," a universe that includes vibrant light and color, spontaneous healing, and encounters with divinity in its many forms. They describe the connection as a core element of sexual relationship, broader, more complex, and more nuanced than the prevailing notion of sex-as-physical-performance, where "function" is health and "dysfunction" is pathology. As a 50-year-old physical therapist from Bozeman, Montana puts it: "I don't have sex–I make love! Big difference. Love is the essence of spirituality. Sex between lovers creates a miracle of intimacy."

The truth is, some women do resist connecting sex and spirit. It is therefore crucial to factor in resistance as one of the complex layers of the spiritual dimensions of women's sexual experience. This paper looks beyond performance definitions and individual pathology to four cultural dynamics in which women's resistance is rooted: selective education, religious belief systems, norms about pleasure, and mind-body separation. Further, it discusses how therapists can challenge these dynamics and find teachable moments to support women's choices for whole-person sex-spirit integration. Information is based on my practice of sex therapy since the mid 1970s and on the nationwide survey I conducted in 1997-8, the first to investigate integrating sexuality and spirituality.

THE ISIS SURVEY ON INTEGRATING SEXUALITY AND SPIRITUALITY

Although some 700 sex surveys were conducted in the twentieth century, most of these focused on intercourse, orgasm, performance, and gender stereotypes (Eriksen, 1998, 1999). None of these surveys focused on issues such as sensitivity, love, intimacy, self-esteem, relationship, commitment, spirituality, safety, empathy, and communication. Yet feminist clinicians universally agree these issues are crucial to women's sexual pleasure and satisfaction (e.g., Kitzinger, 1983; Espin, 1987; Tiefer, 1995; Daniluk, 1998; Ogden, 1999; Savage 1999; Ellison, 2000; Kleinplatz, 2001; Foley, Kope, & Sugrue, 2002). Even the most methodologically revered sex surveys, from the massive *Kinsey Reports* of 1948 (on male sexual behavior) and 1953 (on female sexual behavior) to the 1994 survey of American attitudes, *The Social Organization of Sexuality* never focused on the spiritual meanings of sex. Indeed, they rarely touched on the emotional issues (Eriksen, 1999).

These omissions trouble me because they represent exactly the issues women bring into my therapy sessions and workshops. To broaden my base of observation, I conducted a survey to explore spirituality as an integral factor in sexual response and sexual relationships (Ogden, 1998, 1999a, 2002). The survey appears at the end of this paper.

The survey is titled "Integrating Sexuality and Spirituality." When I was seeking a shorthand for a book on the results, I found the acronym "ISIS"–the name of the most widely worshipped goddess in recorded history, and an uncanny match for this project. Her story goes that she wandered the corners of the earth gathering up the parts of her husband, Osiris, who had been hacked to bits and scattered far and wide by his power-crazed brother. Isis was able to recover all the pieces except his penis. Undaunted, she created a penis out of clay, breathed Osiris back to life, and conceived his child. Since the spirit of this survey is about searching out our missing sexual pieces and putting them together in creative ways, it seemed fitting to invoke the name of Isis, and to ask for her guidance in the service of integrating sex and spirit for women today.

The ISIS methodology is described in detail elsewhere (Ogden, 2002), but let me touch on some highlights here to give context for this paper. The survey questions all came directly from my clinical practice–from the women who had trusted me with their life stories. There were 3,810 responses to the survey, (82 percent of them from women), which places ISIS among the largest sex surveys of the U.S. I obtained about a third of these responses myself or through colleagues, by handing printed questionnaires to groups that are known to have divergent views on both sexuality and spirituality. Such groups included Catholic, Methodist, Mormon, and Unitarian Universalist clergy; students of sexology, family therapy, and theology; nurses, social workers, sex therapists, and other health professionals; sexual abuse survivors, incarcerated male and female sex offenders, lesbian, gay, bisexual, and transgendered individuals, sex workers, and homemakers. The other two-thirds of the responses came as a result of the questionnaire appearing in *New Age* magazine–now titled *Body and Soul* (January-February 1998), and *New Woman* magazine (July 1998).

The ISIS sample is clearly not representative of all Americans. It is nonetheless diverse and inclusive, even beyond the disparity of the groups mentioned above. Women's ages range over seven decades, from 18 to 86. Their geographical locations include every state in America and two Canadian provinces. Most women are Caucasian, but 18 percent are multi-ethnic, African-American, Latina, Native-American, or Asian-American. The women practice twenty-two religious faiths; 71 percent were born Catholics or Protestants, though only 37 percent continue to practice those religions. Almost two-thirds of the women have college degrees, but their socio-economic diversity is broad, including students, laborers, white-collar workers, and professionals. In terms of political affiliation, 58 percent describe themselves as liberal and 80 percent as pro-choice, while about 15 percent describe themselves as conservative and anti-abortion. Eleven percent are bisexual or lesbian and the rest are heterosexual.

Although the questionnaire required no narrative replies, 1,465 respondents sent letters describing how they experienced sexuality and spirituality–an astonishing body of new information on an underreported subject. The ISIS responses provide many teachable moments for clinicians, and this is the spirit in which I offer them here.

One interesting ISIS finding is that even among thousands of women who said they connected sexuality and spirituality, many also wrote about resisting this connection. Nine percent of ISIS women indicated that sex seldom or never needed a spiritual element to be satisfying, and many more acknowledged experiencing guilt, shame, fear, and other disturbing feelings in connection with sex. These feelings were often associated with abuse or violence, which women indicated were violations of their spirits as well as their bodies. More than a quarter of ISIS women reported sexual abuse in childhood or as an adult. This percent is roughly comparable to estimates of the U.S. national average. That said, it must be acknowledged that statistics on sexual abuse are notoriously difficult to gather–perhaps underreported because of the stigma of sexual abuse, and perhaps overreported because there is no universally agreed-upon definition of sexual abuse (Finkelhor, 1994; Ogden, 2002a). The U.S. Census reports no figure for sexual abuse (US Census 2000: http://censtats.census.gov/data/US/01000.pdf.).

Most often, though, ISIS women said their resistance to connecting sex and spirit was due to negative experiences with their partners–husbands, lovers, affairs, one-night stands. They cited man-on-top performance standards that could not be accurately labeled "abuse," but that nonetheless engendered boredom, pain, humiliation, and despair instead of joy and connection. Such resistance was fueled by lack of information, religious proscriptions, pleasure anxiety, and separation of mind, body, emotions, and spirit. In fact, no matter how compellingly most ISIS women stated the case for integrating sex and spirit, mainstream norms such as these regularly undercut their experiences and provided arguments for dis-integration.

ISIS WOMEN BY THE NUMBERS RESISTANCE TO CONNECTING SEX AND SPIRIT

32% said sexual desire had been a source of guilt
28% said their bodies had been a source of shame
15% said they had never thought of spirituality as a part of sex before filling out the survey
9% said it seemed sacrilegious to talk about sex and spirituality together
9% said sex seldom or never needed a spiritual element to be satisfying

ISIS WOMEN SAID THEIR RESISTANCE TO CONNECTING SEX AND SPIRIT WAS BASED ON:

- Fear
- Denial
- Doubt
- Shame
- Guilt
- Judgment
- Numbness
- Good-girl/ bad-girl dichotomies
- Lack of information
- Separation of body and spirit, body and mind
- Pleasure anxiety
- Abdication of responsibility for self
- Over-responsibility for other

THE INFORMATION GAP:
KEEPING SEX AND SPIRIT IN THE DARK

ISIS women reported crucial information gaps that they said created a kind of gaslight syndrome–so gradually depriving them of light that they didn't recognize they were functioning in the dark. Some wrote that they hadn't known all the physiological facts of sex, let alone the emotional and spiritual aspects. Some said they'd been unaware of double standards involved in love, commitment, and partnership. Others wrote of being utterly confused when relational goalposts had shifted without their consent. These ISIS women were well educated–more than two-thirds were college graduates or higher. So why did they lack information about something as basic to their lives as sexual partnership? Perhaps the problem is with our educational system rather than these ISIS women. Few schools and colleges offer opportunities for comprehensive sex education, let alone information about sex and spirit. Sex researchers as long ago as Kinsey have pointed out that higher education doesn't necessarily lead to more sexual knowledge (Kinsey et al., 1948, 1953).

In fact, Western culture has long discouraged women from pursuing any self-knowledge, especially about sex (Heyward, 1989; Brock & Parker, 2001). Even though there has been an explosion of explicit sexual materials since the early 1970s, much of this material is male defined, and little is focused on how to connect sexuality and spirituality. The result is that "good-girl" rules accrete like barnacles to the overall belief that women should be kept uninformed (Ehrenreich, Hess, & Jacobs, 1986, Tavris, 1992, Tiefer & Kaschak, 2001). Reinforced by religion, medicine, and male-dominated sex-survey data, these rules have helped separate sexuality from spirituality and marginalize women's sexual options.

For some of my women therapy clients, for instance, such written and unwritten rules have represented a cruel Sophie's choice, forcing them to give up a portion of what is most precious to their sexual and spiritual growth. One woman complained that her husband was a totally boring lover albeit a caring provider and wonderful father whom she had no intention of leaving. Her physical hunger led to an affair–it was discreet but tortured because of her Catholic guilt and her loyalties to her husband and family. She saw her impossible choice as either to quit seeing her lover cold turkey or to leave her husband and child. Another woman spoke of hot lusty sex, but with a man who was terrified of intimacy and commitment, which left her feeling heartbroken and abandoned when she wasn't with him. Her impossible choice was to break up with the sexiest lover she's ever known or keep "eating her heart out, piece by piece." A lesbian client had to choose between her partner and the Baptist church that was the center of her family's social life, and which preached that homosexuality is inspired by the devil.

What are these women to do? When they separate sex from their spiritual longings they disown a large part of their sexual reality–the paradoxical, generative, life-affirming fullness of their experience. Women who long for more and more meaningful sexual connection with their male partners may risk being seen as a threat because they have tapped into age-old mystery and power. Women who break societal rules (by having an affair or a lesbian lover) may risk shame and rejection, maybe even excommunication. Untenable choices like these typify the sexual quandaries faced by many women today, not only ISIS respondents. No wonder some of us say no to connecting sex and spirit–and no to any sex at all.

A 35-year-old West Virginia college professor summed up the dilemma of experiencing sex "in the light" (or in the know). For many years she assumed that sex and spirit were separate and even antithetical to one another, and when she finally did connect them she was plunged into a kind of cognitive dissonance driven by deep fear. But this woman also demonstrated the courage to change. She sought information from a colleague with a different belief system so that she could broaden her perspective.

> When it (this spiritual sex) first occurred I could not believe it! I know that I was experiencing something that most of the people, if not all of the people, in my [Charismatic/Pentecostal Christian] world had not experienced. I was terrified. After speaking with a friend . . . in the Eastern religions, I understood and did not fear it.

As it turned out, her partner was unable to deal with this influx of spirit or even discuss it with her: "I believe it scared him. Really." This spelled the beginning of the end of the sexual relationship between them. But even without physical sex, she went on to write, a "really intense connection" with this man remains. "Spiritual sex has literally been the most bonding experience, emotionally, psychologically, and sexually of my life."

Her letter illustrates an important point for women who wish to find more spiritual connection in their sexual experience: It may take more than wishing. It may require a commitment to reexamine deeply held beliefs. It may require the information and support necessary to learn new ways of thinking and being. It may mean breaking some of the sexual rules they grew up with and creating new ones. Most certainly it requires the courage to surrender to the often-overwhelming feelings when sex and spirit do connect. Many ISIS respondents agreed that this degree of dedication is special. "Not every person is emotionally or mentally equipped to deal with that intense spiritual attachment," wrote an artist from Santa Monica, California, who spoke wistfully of a long-ago love. She ended on a hopeful note, however: "I am a fearless person . . . and when I fall in love again I refuse to deny myself what I felt that night. The search is now on for a spiritual-based partner who will go to that sacred place with me again."

From these communications from ISIS participants and my therapy clients, I've learned that part of the art of clinical practice concerns timing: honing your ability to sense when a client is ready to opt for positive change. Strike too soon and the agenda becomes yours. Your client may try to move forward, but primarily to please you–because she feels *you* feel she ought to (we've all been there, probably as clients as well as therapists). But let the moment pass and she may retreat into her old constricting habits. A therapist who listens with an open heart as well as an open mind is most likely to be able to recognize that all-important moment of: "Just right." These are the kinds of clinical choice points that become personal growth points for us as well as our clients, for we can best help women face their confounders and demons once we've faced at least some of our own.

RELIGIOUS PROSCRIPTIONS:
THE "MADONNA-WHORE" DICHOTOMY

Religious beliefs also kept ISIS women from connecting sexuality and spirituality or even imagining sex as anything more than physical. "Sex is not spiritual for me, but I want it to be!" wrote a 50-year-old former Catholic, who found that it was impossible for her to reconcile being "good" with also being sexual. Her ideological struggle centered on the socio-religious value placed on the Madonna aspect of sex: virginity and sexual abstinence–a subject about which much has been written (Francoeur, Cornog, & Perper, 1999, Boston Women's Health Book Collective, 2005). She felt that any sexual activity at all caused her to fall far short of this ideal–a blemished Eve cast out of the blessed garden. A 30-year-old former Jehovah's Witness from Lomita, California, reported that she, too, had had no "spiritual sexual experiences." She could allow herself to imagine the possibilities, however. What she envisioned was very different from the black-and-white choice of Madonna or whore:

> The thought of touching a man's (or woman's) soul during sex is so beautiful to me. That in one precious act you could touch an abstract, share a sacred portion of your lover. That to me would make life worth living.

But this woman, too, went on to express deep ambivalence, admitting that she felt like a rebellious child for even thinking sexual relationship might be holy. Yet she also acknowledged that she was in the process of making a radical life shift–changing her religion to the more permissive United Universalist faith so she could allow herself the moral leeway to enjoy sex. "I am trying to embrace the fact that affection is a human need," she wrote, "and the last time I checked, I was in fact human."

Some ISIS women described lifelong struggles with their religious beliefs about sex and spirit. Many had spent years flagellating themselves with negative judgments. A "deeply religious" 26-year-old actor from Norfolk, Virginia reported her inner dialogue:

> Although part of me knows that my sexuality is sacred, another part of me believes that it is not. This part of me makes me feel guilty when my partner gives me pleasure and I don't reciprocate. It also inhibits my exploration of less traditional sex. I am trying to slowly let go of the belief that my sexuality is bad or shameful.

She also wrote of her history of abuse, which she said contributed to her shame and to her resistance to connecting sexuality and spirituality–even though she knew that connection might be what could restore balance to her life.

> Having been sexually abused as a child has hugely affected my sexuality although it is not always clear how. Spiritual sex is one thing that heals those wounds.

This woman speaks for many clients in my practice whose religious training stifles their sexual desire and leads them away from exactly the kind of relational richness they crave. This woman is on the cusp of change. It's important for clinicians to encourage disclosures of this kind and recognize them as teachable moments. There are plentiful opportunities here to help clients say what they want and guide them to articulate their own sexual value systems as distinct from traditional doctrines that limit sexual thought and behavior, and especially limit them for women (Daly, 1978; Heyward, 1989, Hunt, 2000).

CULTURAL RULES:
PLEASURE ANXIETY–THE FEAR OF FEELING GOOD

Even more pervasive than religious proscriptions are the sex-spirit dualities built into the entire culture–including medicine, politics, and the media. "Good-girl" and "bad-girl" are even more pervasive labels than Madonna and Whore. "Good" means purity and moral goodness. It also connotes health and sanity. "Bad" means physical pleasure, with its legendary excesses and dangers–and its perennial fascination. Given no middle ground, it can be terrifying for women to opt for feeling good instead of acting good. Wilhelm Reich, the founder of bioenergetic therapy, recognized this fear and labeled it "pleasure anxiety" (Reich, 1942). He saw this condition widespread in his native Germany in the fascist 1930s and in America during the 1940s and 50s. He argued that families and other social institutions tend to function as "factories of repression"–that is, training grounds for sexual dysfunction, disconnection, joylessness, and violence, especially toward women.

According to the Reichian notion of pleasure anxiety, the prospect of deeply nurturing sexual pleasure may be even more frightening than the prospect of rejection and pain. Pleasure anxiety may manifest as fear of losing control or of feeling dangerously vulnerable. Or it may manifest perversely, as lack of desire or not feeling like a good enough lover. Sexual pleasure may restimulate memories of abuse that contained any element of excitement, warmth, or connection (Miller, 1981; Bass & Davis,1988; Maltz, 1992). Pleasure anxiety may undermine intimacy and commitment, especially for women who have been socialized to caretake and nurture to the exclusion of their own needs (Ogden, 1999). Here, the pleasures of sexual intimacy may even assume a sinister aspect–the specter of falling into the yawning chasm of codependent self-loss (Daly, 1978).

To cope with such fears–or perhaps bypass them without ever fully acknowledging them–many women who enter my practice have developed the fine art of sexual gatekeeping. They become adept at stopping the flow of feeling and energy before it overwhelms them. Some are quick to blame themselves for their sexual inadequacies and dysfunctions. All these defensive maneuvers are well illustrated by a 61-year-old ISIS respondent from Kootenai, Idaho, who wrote of internal blocks for which she chided herself rather than the culture: "I've had orgasms and I've felt intense pleasure, but I'm never totally unaware. Nor totally connected. Part of me hangs back from everything and everyone." Her self-described inability to absorb herself in sexual experience may indeed derive from her personal history as a survivor of multiple sexual abuses. But as Reich observed, the inability to fully embrace sexual pleasure is endemic in a culture that presents sex as dirty and sinful, and that assigns bad-girl names to women who openly enjoy sex. I learned this at every level of the media when the first edition of my book *Women Who Love Sex* was published in 1994. Although the book is based on my clinical research on how women experience sexual pleasure, most interviewers had difficulty saying the title without a nervous giggle or a snide innuendo (one of the most egregious was: "What is this, some kind of phone book?").

Understanding the cultural base of why and how women fear pleasure gives clinicians a broad and potentially powerful perspective. It allows us to look beyond individual pathology to a more useful way of relating to our clients' distress. For instance, from this vantage point we can see that pleasure anxiety is quite "normal," in the sense that so many women suffer from it. Voicing this observation can help women normalize their fears–not minimize them, but at least put them in context.

This broader view also gives us a prime opportunity to educate and encourage clients by eliciting more of their positive story. For instance we can inquire if resisting sex and spirit may have been a crucial survival mechanism even if it no longer serves a useful purpose. We can also offer positive reframes, when appropriate. I might say, for example: "The story you tell about being so scared of feeling good doesn't say to me that there's something intrinsically wrong with you. In fact, it says you're right in the middle of normal. You're responding like any well-socialized woman in this culture–doing what's expected of you, and doing it very well." This kind of therapeutic response can help remove the twin stigmas of "different" and "dysfunctional." It can also ally client with the therapist, along with a vast community of her own peers.

Once your client gets the message that she's not sick and she's not bad and she's not alone, she's hopefully ready to do her work. By broadening the horizon, you allow a new scene to unfold. Now you can begin the job of helping her claim the idea of sexual pleasure on her own terms–what she believes, what she wants, and what spiritual values she experiences in sexual pleasure.

MIND-BODY SEPARATION: ERODING SELF-TRUST

The fear of feeling good may be culturally induced, but it can act systemically on each of us, like a psychospiritual autoimmune disease that fragments body, mind, and spirit. The sexual fragmentation that results can't be cured by conventional allopathic means–the creams, gels, and pills prescribed as if penis-vagina intercourse is the only route to sexual pleasure. But the ravages of fear and fragmentation are well known to practitioners of holistic and integrative medicine, who assert that mind-body separation and resistance to full body-and-soul pleasure can result in all sorts of sex and relationship problems (e.g., Northrup, 1995, 2001). These may include any of the so-called sexual dysfunctions, from low desire to inhibited arousal and orgasm. The good news is that by moving beyond resistance and connecting with pleasure, remarkable incidents of spontaneous healing have proved possible.

Just such a healing was described by an ISIS respondent, a 43-year-old photographer from Des Moines, Iowa, who wrote that her chronic heart condition completely disappeared after she connected sexual and spiritual experience for the first time. Quite literally, she experienced a "change of heart" when she moved from what she named the "coldness" of her former husband to the warm attentions of a high school sweetheart who resurfaced in her life at a crucial moment, and who touched her heart and soul.

Equally interesting is how she explained her reluctance to reveal this encounter: "For years I have lived with not telling anyone about my sex-spirit experience, because I never heard anyone talk about [experiences like] it and was afraid people would think I was crazy." She reported that she felt "crazy" even during the experience, although paradoxically also felt "completely safe." This is a prime moment for therapeutic intervention. Were I her therapist, my Gestalt training would prevail at this point–I might ask her to exaggerate her feelings of both craziness and safety so that she could understand them more clearly. I might also call upon my training in pyschosynthesis–a transpersonal psychology that includes integration of subpersonalities in order to activate the will. Here, I might ask her to converse with the part of her that felt crazy and the part of her that felt safe–to see where those voices originated, which felt stronger, and which she felt most like listening to.

But she didn't consult a therapist. She kept her story secret until she opened *New Age* magazine and read the ISIS questionnaire. Only then did she feel permission to reveal the details of this transformative encounter with her old boyfriend, albeit anonymously. It's significant to me that this was a sexual experience without intercourse—as this presents another teachable moment about the vast spectrum of satisfying sexual experience open to women. It was, in her words, "something better than sex."

> He talked to me all night long, relaxing me, holding me, looking into my eyes. He said we didn't need to have sex. There was something better. He taught me . . . I don't know what to call it. I felt completely safe, floating, saw lights, felt the spirituality. I thought I was going crazy. It felt incredibly great, but scary. My heart problem just went away, the EKG was totally different. The doctors didn't know why. I did, but couldn't tell them. I was too embarrassed to tell anyone.

A caveat to therapists everywhere: Women who are not crazy and fear they are crazy deserve to be: (a) heard out completely and (b) reassured that they're not crazy. A primary role of the therapist is to create a safe environment in which women can tell their stories and voice their fears. Another primary role for us is to think beyond rigid definitions of health and sexual health, whether these come from the DSM or morality-based religious texts. The protestant text I was raised with had me intoning as a teenager: "I have followed the devices and desires of my own heart and there is no health in me." I try to turn this message around in my therapy practice, where most of the women I see ultimately enter therapy to discover (or re-discover) their heart's desires and learn how to follow them. When you open your own heart and your mind, your clients can open theirs, too. Call it countertransference or codependency, it's also a blueprint for transformation.

MOVING BEYOND RESISTANCE TO SEX AND SPIRIT— GENTLE GUIDELINES FOR THERAPISTS

Despite divisive pulls from religion, culture, and reductionist scientific methods, some ISIS respondents reported enormous relief and joy in moving beyond their resistance to connecting sex and spirit. A woman from Israel described the sense of letting go, of surrendering to that connection. She wrote of the resiliency required to make this difficult choice again and again:

> There have been numerous times when my strong spiritual nature has battled with my equally strong sexuality. However, when they combine during love my spirit soars, often leaving me with an intense

joy that my body cannot always contain. Spontaneous tears of deep, pure emotion come forth–much akin to the tears of over-whelming spiritual joy at my children's births.

As this woman eloquently states, the rewards of moving through re-sistance to integrate sex and spirit are enormous. The rewards are also great for the therapist who is privileged to midwife and witness this kind of movement. Here are guidelines I've found useful in helping women move along the path.

The first guideline concerns sex: Understand that sexual experience is much more than intercourse–it includes love, romance, and mystical union as well as physical sensation. Expand your sex history taking to include spiritual needs and dilemmas. Bear in mind that what looks like sexual dysfunction may be social dysfunction rather than individual pa-thology–in which case, DSM definitions and pharmaceutical interven-tions won't help you or your client. The clearer you feel about your own sexual issues, the clearer you can be about guiding your clients through their resistance to connecting sex and spirit. Sex therapy training and supervision can increase your comfort in assessing and confronting your clients' sexual issues. (You can obtain information from the Amer-ican Association of Sex Educators, Counselors, and Therapists, at AASECT.org.)

The next guideline concerns spirit. Understand that spirituality can be very different from religion. Spirituality is rooted in personal and in-dividual inspiration and "knowing." Religion is rooted in cultural be-liefs, traditions, and rituals. Clients may have as much anxiety about spiritual experience as they have about sexual experience, because they may have no frame of reference for it. Whatever your religious convic-tions, the clearer you are about your own spiritual path, the more per-mission your clients will feel to explore and honor theirs. Just because we can't back up our spiritual experiences with statistics doesn't mean they don't exist. I love that Carl Jung calls them "the irrational facts of experience."

Saving best until last, the final guideline concerns women: Listen to women's stories heart-to-heart as well as mind-to-mind. Believe what women tell you is going on in their lives. You may be the first person who ever has. And this kind of listening works both ways. I can say with con-viction: Everything important I've learned about being a therapist I've learned from listening to women. Following is the ISIS Questionnaire. Feel free to use it to elicit stories from women–and feel free to add areas of questioning you think should be included.

INTEGRATING SEXUALITY AND SPIRITUALITY
--A Survey-- © 1997

This is the first survey to inquire about how we integrate sexuality and spirituality, and your participation is extremely valuable. Since each person's experiences are unique, there are no right or wrong answers. You are invited to add your personal statements at the end. If this survey raises uncomfortable feelings, please write them down, even if you do not complete the survey. All the information you provide will remain anonymous. It will be used to educate and inform others. With many thanks for your participation. Gina Ogden, Ph.D., Lic. Marriage and Family Therapist, Cert. Sex Therapist

FIRST, PLEASE TELL US SOMETHING ABOUT YOURSELF: Check the alternatives that best describe your experience, adding whatever information may be necessary.

1. Age _____ Gender: Female ☐ Male ☐ Crossgender ☐ Occupation _____

2. Area you live in (please write first 3 digits of ZIP code) _____

3. Highest education completed 1 Grade School ☐ 2 High School ☐ 3 College ☐ 4 Masters ☐ 5 Doctorate ☐ 6 Post Doctorate ☐

4. Ethnic identification (check all that apply) 1 Caucasian (White) ☐ 2 African-American (Black) ☐ 3 Hispanic ☐ 4 Native American ☐ 5 Asian ☐ 6 Other ☐ (please specify) _____

5. Yearly household income (round numbers) $_____

6. Religion you grew up with 1 Roman Catholic ☐ 2 Protestant ☐ 3 Fundamentalist Christian ☐ 4 Jewish ☐ 5 Buddhist ☐ 6 Mormon ☐ 7 Atheist ☐ 8 Agnostic ☐ 9 None ☐ 10 Other ☐ (please specify) _____

7. Religious affiliation now 1 Roman Catholic ☐ 2 Protestant ☐ 3 Fundamentalist Christian ☐ 4 Jewish ☐ 5 Buddhist ☐ 6 Mormon ☐ 7 Atheist ☐ 8 Agnostic ☐ 9 None ☐ 10 Other ☐ (please specify) _____

8. Political philosophy 1 Liberal ☐ 2 Conservative ☐ 3 Other ☐ (please specify) _____

9. Attitude toward abortion 1 Pro Choice ☐ 2 Anti-Abortion ☐ 3 Other ☐ (please specify) _____

10. Sexual Preference 1 Heterosexual ☐ 2 Bisexual ☐ 3 Lesbian/gay ☐ 4 Other ☐ (please specify) _____

11. Relationship status 1 No current partner ☐ 2 Married ☐ 3 In a committed relationship ☐ 4 Separated ☐ 5 Divorced ☐ 6 Widowed ☐ 7 Other ☐ (please specify) _____

12. Number of years (or fraction of years) with current partner _____

13. Gender of current partner 1 Male ☐ 2 Female ☐ 3 Crossgender ☐

14. Disabilities/chronic illnesses 1 Cancer ☐ 2 Heart Disease ☐ 3 HIV/AIDS ☐ 4 Diabetes ☐ 5 Arthritis ☐ 6 Depression ☐ 7 None ☐ 8 Other ☐ (please specify) _____

15. Experience of sexual abuse 1 As a child ☐ 2 As an adult ☐ 3 Never ☐

16. Addictive use of alcohol and/or drugs 1 In the past ☐ 2 In the present ☐ 3 Never ☐

17. Here are some comments people have made about sex and spirituality. Check *all* that reflect your experience.
   1 ☐ "Sex usually means intercourse."
   2 ☐ "For me, sex is much more than intercourse; it involves all of me--body, mind, heart, and soul."
   3 ☐ "I associate spirituality mainly with going to church."
   4 ☐ "When I open myself to warmth, desire, depth, expansion, and trust, there is no separation between sex and spirit."
   5 ☐ "Sex is for conceiving babies and has little to do with spirituality."
   6 ☐ "It's through my senses that I often experience God."
   7 ☐ "All my life I've been told that people who love sex *too much* will go to hell."
   8 ☐ "Mainly, sex means connection with my partner."
   9 ☐ "Sex is physical, but it also involves love, romance, even mystical union."

10 ☐ "For people who have been sexually disappointed or hurt, consciously giving and receiving sexual pleasure can be healing."

2.

**18. Sexual romance and religious worship
have many kinds of symbols and rituals in common.**
(check *all* that you associate with
both your sexuality *and* your spirituality)

1 ☐ Candles   7 ☐ Special foods
2 ☐ Incense   8 ☐ Words of comfort
3 ☐ Flowers   9 ☐ Words of love
4 ☐ Wine   10 ☐ Laying on of hands
5 ☐ Music   11 ☐ None of the above
6 ☐ Dancing   12 ☐ Other (please specify_____

**19. When I use the word "spirituality" in the
context of my sexuality, I mean:** (check one)

1 ☐ Spirituality but not religion
2 ☐ Religion but not spirituality
3 ☐ Spirituality and religion combined
4 ☐ Other (please specify)_____

**20. To me, it seems sacrilegious to talk about sex and spirituality
together** 1 Yes ☐ 2 No ☐

21. What do sexuality and spirituality involve in your life?
(For each pair of statements, check line segment closest to statement
that best reflects your experience)

Sexuality Involves

1 Excitement	___ ___ ___ ___ ___	Boredom
2 Honesty	___ ___ ___ ___ ___	Deception
3 Caring for others	___ ___ ___ ___ ___	Caring for self
4 Numbed senses	___ ___ ___ ___ ___	Heightened senses
5 Intense body pleasure	___ ___ ___ ___ ___	Minimal body pleasure
6 Intense inner vitality	___ ___ ___ ___ ___	Minimal inner vitality
7 Constraint	___ ___ ___ ___ ___	Liberation
8 Integration	___ ___ ___ ___ ___	Fragmentation
9 Oneness with self	___ ___ ___ ___ ___	Distance from self
10 Oneness with partner	___ ___ ___ ___ ___	Distance from partner
11 Oneness with a power greater than self	___ ___ ___ ___ ___	Distance from a power greater than self
12 Worship	___ ___ ___ ___ ___	Blasphemy
13 Other (please specify)	_____	

Spirituality Involves

14 Excitement	___ ___ ___ ___ ___	Boredom
15 Honesty	___ ___ ___ ___ ___	Deception
16 Caring for others	___ ___ ___ ___ ___	Caring for self
17 Numbed senses	___ ___ ___ ___ ___	Heightened senses
18 Intense body pleasure	___ ___ ___ ___ ___	Minimal body pleasure
19 Intense inner vitality	___ ___ ___ ___ ___	Minimal inner vitality
20 Constraint	___ ___ ___ ___ ___	Liberation
21 Integration	___ ___ ___ ___ ___	Fragmentation
22 Oneness with self	___ ___ ___ ___ ___	Distance from self
23 Oneness with partner	___ ___ ___ ___ ___	Distance from partner
24 Oneness with a power greater than self	___ ___ ___ ___ ___	Distance from a power greater than self
25 Worship	___ ___ ___ ___ ___	Blasphemy
26 Other (please specify)	_____	

22. Which *one* of the above statements would you say is *most* true:

(1) of your current SEXUAL experience? _____

(2) of your current SPIRITUAL experience? _____

**23. Sex needs to have a spiritual element to be
really satisfying.** (check one)

1 ☐ Always true for me
2 ☐ Sometimes true for me
3 ☐ Neither true nor untrue for me
4 ☐ Seldom true for me
5 ☐ Never true for me

**24. With which of the following has sex been a
spiritual experience for you?** (check *all* that apply)

1 ☐ Husband
2 ☐ Wife
3 ☐ Committed partner
4 ☐ Casual encounter
5 ☐ Affair while committed to someone else
6 ☐ Self
7 ☐ None of the above
8 ☐ Other (please specify)_____

**25. Sex has been *most* spiritual with which partner
in Question 24?** (write in number)_____

**26. Sex has been *least* spiritual with which partner
in Question 24?** (write in number)_____

**27. Which of the following have contributed to sex being
a spiritual experience for you?** (check *all* that apply)

1 ☐ Being in love
2 ☐ Conceiving a baby
3 ☐ Being pregnant
4 ☐ Having no fear of getting pregnant
5 ☐ Feeling committed to my partner
6 ☐ Feeling free of responsibility to my partner
7 ☐ Feeling safe
8 ☐ Experiencing a personal crisis
9 ☐ Feeling in control
10 ☐ Feeling controlled
11 ☐ Being in the mood
12 ☐ Aggressive thrusting
13 ☐ Danger
14 ☐ Drinking or drugs
15 ☐ None of the above
16 ☐ Other (please specify)_____

**28. Which *one* of the above circumstances has contributed
most to spiritual sex?** (write in number)_____

**29. Which *one* of the above circumstances has contributed
least to spiritual sex?** (write in number)_____

30. Which of the following have you done to help bring a spiritual dimension to your sexual experiences? (check *all* that apply)

1 ❑ Made eye contact with my partner
2 ❑ Shared deep feelings with my partner
3 ❑ Lit candles or incense
4 ❑ Bathed
5 ❑ Enjoyed special foods
6 ❑ Meditated before getting physical
7 ❑ Made love in a special place
8 ❑ Touched reverently

9 ❑ Kissed soulfully
10 ❑ Played music
11 ❑ Danced
12 ❑ Fantasized or daydreamed
13 ❑ Laughed together
14 ❑ Let go of control
15 ❑ Did nothing special
16 ❑ Other (please specify)_____

31. Which *one* of the above choices has been *most* helpful in bringing a spiritual dimension to your sexuality?
(write in number)_____

32. Which *one* of the above choices has been *least* helpful in bringing a spiritual dimension to your sexuality?
(write in number)_____

33. How have your spiritual beliefs led you to express your sexuality more fully? (check *all* that apply)

1 ❑ By affirming that love is good in all its forms and expressions
2 ❑ By teaching that making love is holy
3 ❑ By opening me to risk deeper intimacy
4 ❑ By giving me faith when I've felt like running away from pleasure
5 ❑ By sanctioning my feelings of longing and passion
6 ❑ By making the physical part of relationship into a sacrament
7 ❑ Other (please specify)_____

34. How have your spiritual beliefs prevented you from expressing your sexuality as fully as you might? (check *all* that apply)

1 ❑ By giving me the message "good girls don't"
2 ❑ By making sexual desire a source of guilt
3 ❑ By making the body a source of shame
4 ❑ By teaching that sex is not for pleasure, but for procreation (conceiving babies)
5 ❑ By teaching that pleasure is more important for a man than for a woman
6 ❑ By keeping me from exploring sexual taboos
7 ❑ Other (please specify)_____

35. Has anything else in your life prevented you from experiencing a sex-spirit connection? (check *all* that apply)

1 ❑ Childhood abuse
2 ❑ Abuse as an adult
3 ❑ Drinking and/or drug use
4 ❑ Depression and/or anxiety
5 ❑ Physical disabilities
6 ❑ Worry about how I look
7 ❑ Getting older
8 ❑ Not having a partner
17 ❑ Other (please specify)_____

9 ❑ Pregnancy
10 ❑ Parenthood
11 ❑ My partner only thinking about physical kicks
12 ❑ Not loving my partner
13 ❑ My partner not loving me
14 ❑ Sex isn't that interesting to me
15 ❑ Spirituality isn't that interesting to me
16 ❑ I've never thought of spirituality as a part of sex before now

36. Which *one* of the above choices has *most* prevented you from experiencing a sex-spirit connection? (write in number)_____

37. Have you ever experienced sexual ecstasy?   1 Yes ❑   2 No ❑

38. Have you ever experienced spiritual ecstasy?   1 Yes ❑   2 No ❑

4.

39.-40. Some people feel that experiences they associate with sexual satisfaction are similar to experiences they associate with spiritual satisfaction. What do you associate with your sexual satisfaction and/or spiritual satisfaction? (check *all* that apply)

	39. Associate with Sexual Satisfaction	40. Associate with Spiritual Satisfaction
Release of body tension	1 ☐	1 ☐
Release of emotional tension	2 ☐	2 ☐
Heightened senses	3 ☐	3 ☐
Clarity of understanding	4 ☐	4 ☐
Surge of energy	5 ☐	5 ☐
Peace and serenity	6 ☐	6 ☐
Feeling loved and accepted	7 ☐	7 ☐
Feeling loving and accepting	8 ☐	8 ☐
Oneness with self	9 ☐	9 ☐
Oneness with partner	10 ☐	10 ☐
Oneness with nature	11 ☐	11 ☐
Oneness with a power greater than self	12 ☐	12 ☐
Other	13 ☐	13 ☐
(please specify)_____		(please specify)_____

41. Which one of the above experiences is *most* essential to your SEXUAL satisfaction? (write in number) _____

42. Which one of the above experiences is *most* essential to your SPIRITUAL satisfaction? (write in number) _____

43. In a moment of SEXUAL ecstasy have you ever had a sense of experiencing God/Universal energy? 1 Yes ☐ 2 No ☐

44. In a moment of SPIRITUAL ecstasy have you ever felt a surge of sexual energy? 1 Yes ☐ 2 No ☐

45. Please indicate how important the following concepts are for your present life situation (circle numbers below)

	Not at all Important					Extremely Important
1 Sexuality	1	2	3	4	5	6
2 Spirituality	1	2	3	4	5	6
3 Religion	1	2	3	4	5	6

(Optional)
Below or on a separate piece of paper, please tell us more about your sexuality and spirituality. How did you discover that sex can be spiritual? What are your most memorable experiences--by yourself and/or with a partner?

(Optional)
Please *print* your name and phone number below if you are willing to be interviewed by telephone about your sexuality and spirituality. If you consent to an interview, the data will not be associated with your name.

Name_____

Phone number_____

REFERENCES AND SUGGESTED READINGS

Bass, Ellen & Davis, Laura. (1988). *The courage to heal: A guide for women survivors of child sexual abuse.* New York: Harper and Row.

Beattie-Jung, Patricia, Hunt, Mary E., & Balakrishnan, Rhadika (2001). *Good sex: Feminist perspectives from the world's religions.* New Brunswick, N.J.: Rutgers University Press.

Bonheim, Jalaja (1997). *Aphrodite's daughters: Women's sexual stories and the journey of the soul.* New York: Fireside.

Boston Women's Health Book Collective (2005). *Our bodies, ourselves. A new edition for a new era.* New York: Touchstone.

Brock, Rita (1988). *Journeys by heart: A Christology of erotic power.* New York: Crossroad.

Brock, Rita & Parker, Rebecca (2001). *Proverbs of ashes: Violence, redemptive suffering, and the search for what saves us.* Boston: Beacon Press.

Daly, Mary (1978). *Gyn-Ecology: The metaethics of radical feminism.* Boston: Beacon Press.

Daniluk, Judith (1998). *Women's sexuality across the life span.* Binghamton, New York: Guilford Press.

Ehrenreich, Barbara, Hess, Elizabeth, & Jacobs, Gloria (1986). *Remaking love: The feminization of sex.* Garden City, N.Y.: Doubleday.

Eriksen, Julia (1998, May). With enough cases, why do you need statistics? Revisiting Kinsey's methodology. *The Journal of Sex Research. 35*, 2. 132-140.

— (1999). *Kiss and tell: Surveying sex in the twentieth century.* Cambridge, Mass.: Harvard University Press.

Ellison, Carol (2000). *Women's sexualities: Generations of women speak about sexual self acceptance.* Oakland, Calif.: New Harbinger.

Espín, Oliva. (1984). Cultural and historical influences on sexuality in Hispanic/Latina women. In Vance, Carol (Ed.). *Pleasure and danger: Exploring female sexuality.* London: Routledge and Kegan Paul. 149-164.

— (1987). Issues of identity in the psychology of Latina lesbians. In Boston Lesbian Psychologies Collective, *Lesbian psychologies.* Urbana: University of Illinois Press.

— (1997). *Latina realities: Essays on healing, migration, and sexuality.* Boulder, Colo.: Westview Press.

Finkelhor, D., Dzuiba-Leatherman, J. (1994). Children as victims of violence: a national survey. *Pediatrics* 94:413-420.

Foley Sallie, Kope, Sally, & Sugrue, Dennis. (2002). *Sex matters for women: A complete guide to taking care of your sexual self.* Binghamton. New York: Guilford Press.

Francoeur, Robert, Cornog, Martha, & Perper, Timothy (Eds.) (1999). *Sex, love, and marriage in the 21st century: The next sexual revolution.* Lincoln, Nebraska: iUniverse. com, Inc.

Heyward, Carter (1989). *Touching our strength: The erotic as power and the love of God.* New York: Harper Collins.

Hunt, Mary. E. (1991). *Fierce tenderness: A feminist theology of friendship*. New York: Crossroad.

— (2000). Too sexy for words: The changing vocabulary of religious ethics. In Sands, Kathleen (Ed.). *God forbid: Religion and sex in American public life*. New York: Oxford University Press. 155-166.

Kinsey, A. C., Pomeroy, W. B., Martin, C. E., & Gebhard, P. H. (1953). *Sexual behavior in the human female*. Philadelphia: W.B. Saunders Co.

Kinsey, A. C., Pomeroy, W. B., Martin, C. E. (1948). *Sexual behavior in the human male*. Philadelphia: W.B. Saunders Co.

Kitzinger, Sheila (1983). *Woman's experience of sex: The facts and feelings of female sexuality at every stage of life*. New York: Putnam.

Kleinplatz, Peggy J. (Ed.). (2001) *New directions in sex therapy: Innovations and alternatives*. Philadelphia: Brunner-Routledge.

Maltz, Wendy (1992). *The sexual healing journey: A guide for survivors of sexual abuse*. New York: Harper Collins.

Miller, Alice (1981). *The drama of the gifted child*. New York: Basic Books.

Northrup, Christane (1995). *Women's bodies, women's wisdom: Creating physical and emotional health and healing*. New York: Bantam.

— (2001). *The wisdom of menopause: Creating physical and emotional health and healing during the change*. New York: Bantam.

Ogden, Gina (1998, July). How sex can be spiritual. *New Woman*. 105-109.

— (1999). *Women who love sex: An inquiry into the expanding spirit of women's erotic experience*. (Rev. Ed.). Cambridge, Mass.: Womanspirit Press.

— (1999 a, January-February). Sex and spirit: The healing connection. *New Age*. 78-81, 128-130.

— (2001, December). The taming of the screw: Reflections on "A new view of women's sexual problems." *Women and Therapy*. 24, 1&2. 17-21. Simultaneously published in: Tiefer, L. & Kaschak, E. (Eds.). *A New View of Women's Sexual Problems*. Binghamton, New York: Haworth Press. 17-21.

— (2001a). Integrating sexuality and spirituality: A group approach to women's sexual dilemmas. In Kleinplatz, Peggy J. (Ed.). *New directions in sex therapy: Innovations and alternatives*. Philadelphia: Brunner-Routledge. 322-346.

— (2002). Sexuality and spirituality in women's relationships: Preliminary results of an exploratory survey. *Working Paper 405*. Wellesley College Center for Research on Women, Wellesley, Mass.

— (2002a, January). Spiritual dimensions of sex therapy: An integrative approach for women (a continuing education insert). *Contemporary Sexuality*. P.O. Box 5488, Richmond, Virginia: American Association of Sex Educators, Counselors, and Therapists.

— (2002b, May). What do sex surveys *really* tell us? *Sojourner*. 27, 9. 29, 32-33.

— (2006) *The heart and soul of sex: Making the ISIS connection*. Boston: Shambhala.

Reich, Wilhelm (1942). *The function of the orgasm*. New York: Orgone Institute Press (new translation: 1973). New York: Farrar, Straus and Giroux.

Savage, Linda (1999). *Reclaiming goddess sexuality: The power of the feminine way.* Carlsbad, Calif.: Hay House.

Tavris, Carol (1992). *The mismeasure of woman.* New York: Simon and Schuster.

Tiefer, Leonore (1995). *Sex is not a natural act and other essays.* Boulder, CO: Westview Press.

— (2000, August). Sexology and the pharmaceutical industry: The threat of co-optation. *The Journal of Sex Research 37*, 3. 273-283.

Tiefer, Leonore & Kaschak, Ellyn (Eds.). (2001). *A New View of Women's Sexual Problems.* Binghamton, New York: Haworth Press.

Wade, Jenny (2004). *Transcendent sex: When lovemaking opens the veil.* New York: Paraview Pocket Books.

Traditional Religious Doctrine and Women's Sexuality: Reconciling the Contradictions

Judith C. Daniluk

Nicolle Browne

SUMMARY. For many women the connection between sexuality and spirituality is frequently experienced in the context of their past or current religious beliefs–beliefs that privilege intercourse and male pleasure while ignoring much of what is rich and important in women's sexual experiencing–resulting in feelings of shame, guilt and disconnection from a vital source of their power and pleasure. The focus of this paper is on the differences between religiosity and spirituality, and how women can be assisted to develop more positive and affirming sexual self constructions and nurture a more empowering sense of spirituality in their lives, in the face of sometimes oppressive religious teachings and beliefs. Suggestions are provided for helping women create more positive connections between their spiritual and sexual selves, irrespective of their religious affiliations and beliefs.

Judith C. Daniluk, PhD, is Professor of Education and Counseling Psychology and Special Education, University of British Columbia. Nicolle Browne earned her MEd at the University of British Columbia.

INTRODUCTION

When I was approached by the editors about writing an article for this special issue on women's sexuality and spirituality, my first inclination was to decline their request. While intrigued by the topic, I had serious doubts about my ability to write about spiritual issues, much less write something that might contribute to the readership of *Women & Therapy*. Certainly, the issue of spirituality has reared its head in my research and writing related to women's experiences of their sexuality (e.g., Daniluk, 1993; 1998), and spiritual questioning and issues of faith often are an important theme in my work with infertile women as they try to deal with, overcome, and reconcile themselves to their inability to produce a child (Daniluk, 2001; Zeiger, 1995). And there can be little question about the increasing interest in, and attention to, spirituality in the literature in recent years–both feminist and mainstream (e.g., Eisler, 1995; Feuerstein, 2003; Gudorf, 1994; Heyward, 1989; Mahoney & Graci, 1999; Ogden, 2002a and b; Timmerman, 1992). But I do not consider myself a particularly spiritual person, and as a woman who was raised within a devoutly Catholic family (i.e., regular church attendance, communion, confirmation, Catholic elementary and secondary school education), it was, and perhaps still is, impossible to untangle the vestiges and webs of my Catholic upbringing, in terms of the role of my spiritual beliefs in my experience of my sexuality.

In speaking with my co-author about this issue, reviewing the literature on spirituality as we contemplated writing this paper, and in recalling the challenges of so many women I have spoken to and worked with over the years, I realized that I am not alone in this struggle. According to Moore (1980), "Of all the enigmas encountered by man [or woman] during his [her] earthly existence, the relationship between sexuality and spirituality is surely one of the strangest of all mazes" (p. 1). It is fair to say this relationship is likely even more complicated when organized religion is involved–especially for women (Simpson & Ramberg, 1997; Stevens, Caron & Pratt, 2003).

Indeed, spirituality is a difficult construct to define (Burkhardt, 1994; Mahoney & Graci, 1999; Shahabi et al., 2002), being associated so often with traditional, organized religions and religious faith and practices (Ogden, 2002a and b). In her recent survey research of 2667 women and 1143 men, Ogden (2002a and b) noted how for many respondents the connection between their sexuality and their spirituality was frequently experienced in the context of their religious beliefs. Religious teachings provide the framework within which people judge the rightfulness or wrongfulness of their sexual feelings, fantasies, and activities, as well as those of others (Gil, 1990; Hyde, 1994). In a recent survey of 2,039 students between the ages of 18 and 22 years, Stevens et al. (2003) found that the social control function religious values have historically served for young adults still exists. "Those who felt religion played an important role in their lives were much more likely to feel that virginity was important in a life partner, premarital sex was not okay, abortion was unacceptable, and sex without love was not okay" (p. 8).

Although some researchers and writers emphasize the potential for "profound sexual and spiritual encounters" among those holding strong religious beliefs such as practicing Christians (MacKnee, 2002, p. 234), Jung (2000) underscores the tremendous power religions have to maintain negative constructions of women's sexuality in accordance with the values and power of patriarchy. Certainly that has been our experience. With varying degrees of success, I have spent the better part of my adult life attempting to exorcise some of the religious demons related to my gender and sexuality that had firmly taken up residence in my psyche and sexual self-esteem. Even though she was raised a few decades later, during a time when sexual pleasure was the ethos for young women as well as men and reliable birth control was easily accessible, my co-author also struggled to claim a sense of sexual entitlement and integration, often facing stereotypes and judgments based on mainstream religious ethics on what a 'good girl' is despite her not being a member of any particular religious institution.

It would appear that we are not alone in our struggles (Andolsen, 1992; Ogden, 2002a and b; Simpson & Ramberg, 1997). Consequently, the focus of this paper is on how we, as feminists and mental health professionals, can help our women clients develop more positive and affirming sexual self constructions and nurture a more empowering sense of spirituality in their lives, in the face of sometimes oppressive religious teachings and beliefs. We begin by addressing the differences between spirituality and religiosity. We then discuss some of the more dominant religious perspectives regarding women's sexualities and sexual natures as well as the consequences of these beliefs. The paper concludes with suggestions on how we can help our women clients create more positive connections between their spiritual and sexual selves, irrespective of their religious affiliations and beliefs.

SPIRITUALITY DEFINED

What is spirituality and how does it differ from religiosity? Robert Wuthnow (cited in Evans, 2001) traces the shifts in notions of spirituality over the past five decades in North America. He notes how in the 1950's spirituality was very closely tied to belonging to a church or organized religion. However, during the 60's, people started to look outside of what they perceived as the rigid and conservative constraints of church and religious institutions, in an attempt to make meaning of their lives. This shift has led to the more current zeitgeist of a highly personalized spirituality–one that is "personally and variously defined" by individuals (Ogden, 2002a and b, p. 1). This type of spiritual connection and enlightenment might be realized not in a church, but through meditation, nature, art, music, or sexuality.

According to Ogden (2002a and b) even the emerging literature on religion and sexuality is "somewhat misleading" in that it still "tends to equate the notion of religious experience (often culturally and communally defined) with the notion of spiritual experience (often personally defined)" (p. 5). From this perspective, in terms of a distinction, religion is characterized by particular rules and consequences, traditions, and community, while spirituality is characterized by personal and individual inspiration and knowing.

In an effort to distinguish religiosity from spirituality, Mahoney and Graci (1999) sent questionnaires to 22 experts in death studies and 13 experts in spiritual studies. Both groups noted differences between being spiritual versus religious. There was consensus that the meaning of the term spirituality is currently changing. "The themes most strongly associated with spirituality in both groups were charity, community or connectedness, compassion, forgiveness, hope, meaning, and morality" (p. 521). Elkins, Hedstrom, Hughes, Leaf and Saunders (1988) based the development of their "Spiritual Orientation Inventory" to measure the spirituality of those not affiliated with a traditional religion, on dimensions such as the sacredness of life, altruism, idealism, having a life mission, and the search for meaning and purpose in life. While some of these dimensions are embedded within the values of most traditional religions, the authors in both studies emphasize the role of individual perceptions and values in the determination of spirituality for those who are not religious. Alternately, scriptures and religious teachings are critical in the determination of spiritual beliefs and values for those who adhere to traditional religions (Helm, Berecz & Nelson, 2001; Hyde, 1994; Jung, 2000; Strauss, 2001; Simpson & Ramberg, 1997).

The centrality of individual perceptions and beliefs in the experience of spirituality is apparent in much of the recent feminist literature on sexuality and spirituality. Common elements in these notions of the relationship between spirituality and sexuality includes an emphasis on meaning (Daniluk, 1998; Timmerman, 1992), intuition and self love (Bonheim, 1997), oneness with self, partner, or a universal or divine presence (Eisler, 1995), transcendence and transformation (Heyward, 1989), and the erotic as a source of power and healing (Gimbutas, 1989; Lorde, 1994; Shaw, 1994). This is consistent with Burkhardt's (1994) grounded theory investigation into women's understandings of spirituality through in-depth interviews with 12 adult women in Appalachia. For these women, spirituality was experiences as:

> . . . a unifying force permeating all of life, and manifested through one's becoming and connecting . . . Spirituality shapes and gives meaning to life, is expressed in one's being, knowing, and doing, and is experienced within caring connection with self, others, nature, and ultimate other. Spirituality was related to an inner knowing and source of strength. (p.12)

Personal definition, intuitive knowing, and a sense of "connectedness to the whole, or to the universe, or to the divine" (Evans, 2001), appear to be critical in constructions and the experience of spirituality for those who do not adhere to a particular religious doctrine. It follows then, that a spirituality constructed through a personal lens of meaning and values–one based on love, harmony and connectedness to the whole, and guided by an inner knowing–has the potential to open up endless possibilities for vital, woman-affirming and personally empowering sexual self constructions and experiences. Such is not the case, however, for many women whose sexuality and sexual self perceptions are informed and reinforced by religious doctrine.

RELIGIOUS PERSPECTIVES AND CONSEQUENCES

Some highly positive and even relatively neutral perspectives on women's sexuality and sexual nature are promoted by some religious groups. For example, Hinduism's highly positive view of sexuality is supported by *Kama*, one of the four acceptable approaches to life, as reflected in the erotic Kama Sutra (Hyde, 1994). The eastern Tantric traditions within Hinduism and Buddhism also view sexuality as integral to spiritual pursuits and value the principles of sexual equality, sexual intimacy without domination, and reciprocity instead of power relation-ships (Shaw, 1994). Both Eisler (1995) and Bonheim (1997) note the value placed on sexuality as a sacred source of healing the psyche and nurtur-ing the spirit throughout history in cultures such as Egypt and Japan.

However, such positive, woman-affirming perspectives on sexuality are not supported by most religions whose teachings are based on cur-rent interpretations of the Bible, The Torah, or the Qur'an (Hyde, 1994). A thorough review of current Christian, Orthodox Jewish, Catholic, Protestant, or Muslim perspectives on women's sexuality is beyond the scope of this paper. For an in-depth review of these teachings, the reader is referred to Andolsen (1992), Eisler (1995), Gudorf (1994), Jung (2000), Simpson & Ramberg (1997).

Being based upon or interpreted through patriarchal lenses, the com-mon elements related to women's sexuality in the religious teachings mentioned above include: a dualistic separation between mind and body, spirit and sexuality; an emphasis on intercourse and procreation in circumscribing the definition and purpose of sex; valuing and treasur-ing of virginity; insistence on sexual exclusivity between married part-ners; sanctions against sex outside of marriage; and admonishment of masturbation, sexual fantasies, and homosexuality (Helie, 2004; Hyde, 1994; Jung, 2000; Pellauer, 2004; Slowinski, 1997; Simpson & Ramberg, 1997). Jung (2000) notes how the Catholic church teaches that only conjugal coitus is good with the essential elements necessary for the completion of the marital act being penile penetration, release of semi-nal fluid into the vagina, and male pleasure and orgasm but only because these are required for ejaculation. She underscores how "The Catholic emphasis on the perpetual virginity of Mary symbolizes the church's ongoing inability to come to terms with the goodness of female sexual pleasure" (p. 33). With an emphasis on sex for procreation for the purpose of family building, the teachings in Orthodox Judaism oppose sex out-side of marriage and the use of birth control (Zeiger, 1995). In her article entitled "Holy hatred," Helie (2004) notes similarly oppressive views of women's sexuality in the majority of Muslim countries based on inter-pretations of the Qur'an, with several Muslim countries still carrying the death penalty for same sex relationships.

With their emphasis on sexual restraint and sex for procreation, women's capacity for sexual pleasure is neither acknowledged nor affirmed within most traditional religious frameworks (Hyde, 1994; Simpson & Ramberg, 1997). Jung (2000) notes that "there is much cru-elty" hidden deep in the world's moral traditions, with religion pres-cribing a view of women's sexuality that is long on shoulds, duty, and obligation, and very short on pleasure. Current religious discourse regarding women's sexuality privileges intercourse and male pleasure, while ignoring much of what is important in women's sexual experiencing in terms of meaning, love, commitment, intimacy and pleasure, contributes to the silencing of women's realities, and excludes the diversity and range of experiences of not only heterosexual women, but lesbian, bisexual, and transgendered women (Townsend, 2001).

What are the consequences of these oppressive messages for women who were raised from childhood within traditional religious contexts, as well as those whose spirituality in adulthood is informed by their religious beliefs and practices? Indeed, as Wolf (1997) notes, it is very difficult to untangle the organic and social elements in women's sexual experiences. "So integrated are social and biological factors in [all] women's experience of desire and pleasure that it is difficult to tease them apart . . . joy, like its loss, is not only biologically but also culturally grounded" (p. 34) as well as being religiously sustained. How then, do these traditional religious teachings which have been broadly incorporated into our cultural beliefs about sex and sexuality, shape and impact the sexual experiences, identities and sexual self perceptions of girls and women regardless of religious affiliation.

As early as 1953 in their book *Sexual Behavior in the Human Female, Kinsey, Pomeroy, Martin and Gebhard* reported the consistent negative impact of Christianity and Christian teachings on women's capacity for experiencing sexual pleasure. Almost 50 years later, long after the purported sexual revolution of the 60's and 70's, in her 2002 survey Ogden found that participants' attitudes about religion figured heavily in their narratives about their sexual experiences. While some respondents reported that some religious beliefs about sex fostered feelings of love, intimacy, altruism and a sense of oneness with the divine, other beliefs engendered feelings of guilt, shame, fear, sexual paralysis and a separation from self. She quotes one respondent as saying: "Man, Catholicism sure does screw up one's pleasure thoughts" (p. 17). Indeed,

> The absence of sexual joy in so many women's lives is in part a consequence of the way 'good sex' has been constructed in Christian moral traditions. While there is some room for women's sexual delight along the fringes of this sacred canopy, it is not highlighted under the big tent. (Jung, 2000, p. 33)

For many of the women in my sexuality research groups (e.g., Daniluk, 1993), and for many women clients with whom I have worked over the past 25 years, the overwhelming legacy of religious teachings about women's sexuality are often debilitating feelings of shame and guilt (Daniluk, 1998). Women feel shame about their female bodies, especially those parts most associated with their distinct sexuality–their breasts and genitals. They feel shame when menstruation begins–symbolically marking their fertility and entrance into womanhood. And in an ironic paradox, they feel shame when menstruation ceases at menopause–marking the end of their fertility and symbolically the end of their sexual value. They feel shame when their bodies are unable to produce a child–the ultimate goal that legitimizes their female sexuality and their inherent worth in the eyes of God or Allah (Daniluk, 1999; Zeiger, 1995). And they feel guilty for all their sexual thoughts, fantasies, feelings and behaviors that do not fit within the rigid and oppressive constraints advocated within these moral traditions.

According to Gil (1990), there is considerable evidence in the litera-ture that the sexually guilty person is usually one who is devout and constant in their religious beliefs (Gil, 1990). In examining gender dif-ferences in religious fundamentalism, Helm et al. (2001) found that guilt and shame are the common consequence for women, when the 'real' self does not measure up or reflect the ideal sexual self supported by Christian doctrine. Pick, Givaudan and Kline (2005) concur. According to these authors the tension between sexual desire and religious norms leads to limited communications and anxiety related to sexuality, espe-cially for women, with the most common feelings associated with sexual anxiety being "guilt, shame, tension or stress, as well as fear and pres-sure" (p. 45).

Townsend (2001) suggests that "our sexuality is basic to our capacity to know and to experience God" (p. 157). Sexuality and spirituality are complementary, interdependent and inseparable aspects of being fully human. "Present to one another in an open system, they enhance each other. Growth in one facilitates growth in the other as the whole person grows . . . a fully developed spirituality implies a fully developed sexu-ality, and *vice versa*" (Chavez-Garcia & Helminiak, 2004, p. 151). If that is the case, the sad irony for many women is that traditional religious teach-ings leave them to varying degrees guilt-ridden about, ashamed of, and disconnected from their bodies, their sexuality, and their sexual selves, and thereby unable to really know and experience the spiritual aspects of their humanity. How then, can we help our women clients reduce their feelings of shame and guilt related to their sexuality? How can we assist them in embracing a spirituality that affirms and celebrates their sexuality and sexual pleasure, in all its potential richness and diversity, ir-respective of their religious affiliations?

RECONCILING THE CONTRADICTIONS

Sexual script theory (Jones & Hostler, 2001; Simon & Gagnon, 1986) and feminist interactionist perspectives (Daniluk, 1998) are useful theo-retical frames from which to work on these complex issues (Slowinski, 1997). The goal of this work is to first see the client's sexual world through her eyes, to help her gain insight into the beliefs, values and as-sumptions that construct her sexual self perceptions and behaviors, and then to assist her in developing alternate perspectives (scripts) and mean-ings. For example, by examining the messages and beliefs women clients hold about masturbation, and challenging the source of these messages and the validity of these beliefs (e.g., why would the lord create woman with a body part–the clitoris–the only function of which is to provide pleasure, if women were not meant to experience sexual pleasure), they may begin to perceive their sexual pleasure as being consistent with God's will, rather than something "immoral," or "bad," or "sinful."

For those women whose sexuality has been shaped, damaged, and cir-cumscribed by dualistic, oppressive, and restrictive anti-pleasure, anti-woman religious doctrine and beliefs, a first step is to have clients identify the beliefs and assumptions they hold about women's sexuality in general and their sexuality in particular. It is necessary to explore the meanings clients hold related to their sexual self perceptions, their bodies, and the way they feel about and expresses their unique sexualities. In par-ticular, it is important to explore the messages they received while grow-ing up, as well as identifying the social, cultural and religious sources of these messages. We can then begin to assist clients in teasing out and sep-arating the positive, helpful beliefs and assumptions they hold related to faith, morality, and values in general, from the shame- and guilt-inducing messages they have incorporated related to their bodies and their sexuality. The reader is directed to the first author's (Daniluk, 1998) book on women's sexuality for numerous examples of how to identify and chal-lenge the source of negative sexual messages and meanings.

According to Jung (2000), "Recognizing and naming what makes for bad sex is important work, but women must begin to (re)construct their theological and moral traditions offering society new accounts of what makes for good sex" (p. 42). Pellauer (2004) similarly emphasizes how, to correct mistaken and misbegotten notions regarding the nature of women's sexuality "we must create more accurate accounts of female sexuality" (p. 161). Several feminist writers attempt to do just that, by challenging the validity of male defined interpretations of scriptures and religious teachings regarding women's sexuality (e.g., Bonheim, 1997; Eisler, 1995). Consistent with Lorde's (1978, 1994) contention that sexual pleasure can contribute much to a woman's sense of self-love, self-worth, and connection, Jung (2000) presents a Roman Catholic's perspective on women's sexual pleasure and delight, focusing on the recovery and celebration of women's bodily experience and the articulation of a more woman-affirming moral tradition. Christine Gudorf (1994) also uses a Roman Catholic lens to make a persuasive case for the moral goodness of women's sexual pleasure and delight. A pastoral counselor and marriage and family therapist, Townsend (2001) challenges the dualism inherent in Christian doctrine, and presents a more holistic theology of women's sexuality that honors and celebrates the central role of embodied sexuality in women's "capacity to know and experience God" (157). In an attempt to celebrate women's sexuality, Pellauer (2004) focuses on the moral significance of female orgasm, and both Heyward (1989) and Timmerman (1992) articulate emerging feminist theologies that connect the body with personal power and self determination. Sharing these woman-positive, feminist perspectives on the interface between religion, spirituality, and sexuality can be a powerful tool in helping women clients embrace more affirming, integrated and woman-positive views of their sexuality, within the moral, religious, and spiritual traditions that guide the other aspects of their lives.

Readers are also directed to the important work of feminist sexuality therapists who reject the dualistic and value-ladened categories of sexual function and dysfunction, in favor of more expansive and holistic views of women's sexuality that emphasize self-love and acceptance, pleasure, connection, and the wide range of experiences and activities that constitute the diverse sexualities of women (e.g., McCormick, 1994; Ogden, 1999; 2002b; Schwartz & Rutter, 1998; Tiefer & Kaschak, 2001). Current feminist efforts to articulate more expansive, woman-positive, empowering connections between women's sexuality and spirituality can also help clients develop and articulate more affirming connections between their spiritual and sexual selves (e.g., Bonheim, 1977; Gimbutas, 1989; Lorde, 1994; Ogden, 2002 a and b; Shaw, 1994; Timmerman, 1992).

It is also important to recognize that the negative and oppressive beliefs and dominant scripts related to sexuality in general and women's sexuality in particular, like the air we breathe, permeate, and to varying degrees have shaped the lives and experiences of all women–not just those for whom religiosity was or is a part of their lives (Daniluk, 1998). Consequently, it is important that therapists working with clients on issues related to their sexuality and sexual self-perceptions examine our own beliefs, values, and messages regarding the sexual nature, needs, and rights of women, and to be aware of our comfort or discomfort in addressing these issues (Bridges, Lease, & Ellison, 2004). It is necessary for therapists to monitor our reactions to hearing women's narratives about sexuality, spirituality and religiosity, and to be aware of what this triggers for us based on our own upbringing and beliefs–being vigilant to respect and honor each client's world view–irrespective of how these views may conflict with our own values.

Finally, it is important for therapists to acknowledge and appreciate the tremendous challenges women face in turning off the negative, oppressive tapes that have played in their minds and lives for many years and shaped their understanding and experiences of their sexuality. As one woman said to me after a workshop focused on helping women reduce sexual shame and guilt, and create healthier sexual self-constructions: "You need to let people know how hard it is to turn off those tapes and really start to feel good about your body and your sexuality. It doesn't happen overnight. It's an ongoing, lifelong process."

For all women, it is an ongoing challenge to nurture and sustain a spirituality that celebrates women's sexuality and erotic potential in all of its varied forms of expression, within a social and cultural context that so often disregards, diminishes, and disqualifies that potential. However, the rewards for doing so can be great in the form of healing, celebration, passion, pleasure, intimacy, love, and connection with self, others, and the divine. As Pellauer (2004) so aptly states:

> We need to follow the trails of our joy with the same persistent adventurousness with which we have explored the pains of sexual abuses. We need to explore this terrain in a mood that can acknowledge the disappointments without letting go of the delight . . . Celebrating women's sexuality is key to good sexual ethics, feminist or not. Such a celebration requires a many-meaninged, many-valued, many-voiced complexity that can rejoice in the fact that we are many and not one . . . We need many more voices raised to describe, to speculate, to linger over the meaning of our delights. (p. 182)

As feminist therapists, we can play an important role in this celebration, in our own lives, and in our work with our clients.

REFERENCES

Andolsen, B.H. (1992). Whose sexuality? Whose tradition? Women, experience and Roman Catholic sexual ethics. In R.M. Green (Ed.), *Religion and sexual health: Ethical, theological and clinical perspectives* (pp. 55-77). Boston, MA: Dluwer Academic Publishers.

Bonheim, J. (1997). *Aphrodite's daughter's: Women's sexual stories and the journey of the soul.* New York: Fireside.

Bridges, S.K., Lease, S.H., & Ellison, C.R. (2004). Predicting sexual satisfaction in women: Implications for counselor education training. *Journal of Counseling & Development, 82,* 158-166.

Burkhardt, M.A. (1994). Becoming and connecting: Elements of spirituality for women. *Holistic Nursing Practice, 8,* 12-21.

Chavez-Garcia, S., & Helminiak, D.A. (2004). Sexuality and spirituality: Friends, not foes. *Journal of Pastoral Care, 39,* 151-164.

Daniluk, J.C. (2001). *The infertility survival guide: Everything you need to know to cope with the challenges while maintaining your sanity, dignity, and relationships.* Oakland, CA: New Harbinger Publications.

Daniluk, J.C. (1999). When biology isn't destiny: Implications for the sexuality of childless women. *Canadian Journal of Counselling, 33,* 79-94.

Daniluk, J. (1998). *Women's sexuality across the lifespan: Challenging myths, creating meanings.* New York: The Guildford Press.

Daniluk, J. (1993). The meaning and experience of female sexuality. *Psychology of Women Quarterly, 17,* 53-69.

Eisler, R. (1995). *Sacred pleasure: Sex, myth, and the politics of the body.* San Francisco: Harper Collins.

Elkins, D.N., Hedstrom, I.J., Hughes, L.L., Leaf, J.A., & Saunders, C. (1988). Toward a humanistic-phenomenological spirituality: Definition, description, and measurement. *Journal of Humanistic Psychology, 28,* 5-18.

Evans, K. (2001). Journeys of the spirit. *Health, 15,* 118-124.

Feuerstein, G. (2003). *Sacred sexuality.* Rochester: Inner Traditions.

Gil, V.E. (1990). Sexual fantasy experiences and guilt among conservative Christians: An exploratory study. *Journal of Sex Research, 27,* 629-639.

Gimbutas, M. (1989). *The language of the goddess.* San Francisco: Harper & Row.

Gudorf, C.E. (1994). *Body, sex and pleasure.* Cleveland, OH: The Pilgrim Press.

Helie, A. (2004). Holy hatred. *Reproductive Health Matters, 12,* 120-124.

Helm Jr., H.W., Berecz, J.M., & Nelson, E.A. (2001). Religious fundamentalism and gender differences. *Pastoral Psychology, 50,* 25-37.

Heyward, C. (1989). *Touching our strength: The erotic as power and the love of God.* New York: Harper Collins.

Hyde, J.S. (1994). *Understanding human sexuality.* New York: McGraw-Hill.

Jones, S.L., & Hostler, H. (2001). Sexual script theory: An integrative exploration of the possibilities and limits of sexual self-definition. *Journal of Psychology and Theology, 30,* 120-130.

Jung, P.B. (2000). Sexual pleasure: A Roman Catholic perspective on women's delight. *Theology & Sexuality, 12*, 26-47.

Kinsey, A.C., Pomeroy, W.B., Martin C.E., & Gebhard, P.H. (1953). *Sexual behavior in the human female*. Philadelphia: W.B. Saunders.

Lorde, A. (1978). *Uses of the erotic: The erotic as power*. Trumansburg, NY: Out and Out Books/Crossing Press.

Lorde, A. (1994). Uses of the erotic: The erotic as power. In J.B. Nelson & S.P. Longfellow (Eds.), *Sexuality and the sacred: Sources for theological reflection* (pp. 75-79). Louisville, KY: John Knox Press.

MacKnee, C. (2002). Profound sexual and spiritual encounters among practicing Christians: A phenomenological analysis. *Journal of Psychology and Theology, 30*, 234-244.

Mahoney, M.J., & Graci, G.M. (1999). The meanings and correlates of spirituality: Suggestions from an exploratory survey of experts. *Death Studies, 23*, 521-528.

McCormick, N. (1994). *Sexual salvation: Affirming women's rights and pleasures*. Westport Conn.: Praeger.

McIlvenna, T. (1977). *Meditations on the gift of sexuality*. San Francisco: Specific Press.

Moore, J. (1980). *Sexuality and spirituality*. San Francisco: Harper & Row.

Ogden, G. (2002a). *Sexuality and spirituality in women's relationship*. (Wellesley Centers for Women, Working Paper No. 405). Wellesley, MA: Wellesley Centers for Women.

Ogden, G. (2002b). Spiritual dimensions of sex therapy: An integrative approach for Women (a continuing education insert). *Contemporary Sexuality. i-vii*.

Ogden, G. (1999). *Women who love sex: An inquiry into the expanding spirit of women's erotic experience*. Cambridge, MA: Womanspirit Press.

Pellauer, M.D. (2004). The moral significance of female orgasm: Toward sexual ethics that celebrates women's sexuality. *Journal of Feminist Studies in Religion, 9,* 161-182.

Pick, S., Givaudan, M., & Kline, K.F. (2005). Sexual pleasure as a key component of integral sexual health. *Feminism and Psychology, 15*, 44-49.

Schwartz, P., & Rutter, V. (1998). *The gender of sexuality*. Thousand Oaks, CA: Pine Forge Press.

Shahabi, L., Powell, L.H., Musick, M.A., Pargament, K.I., Thoresen, C.E., Williams, D., Underwood, L., Ory, M.A. (2002). Correlates of self-perceptions of spirituality in American adults. *Annals of Behavioral Medicine, 24*, 59-68.

Shaw, M. (1994). *Passionate enlightenment: Women in Tantric Buddhism*. New Jersey: Princeton University Press.

Simon, W., & Gagnon, J.H. (1986). Sexual scripts: Performance and change. *Archives of Sexual Behavior, 15*, 97-120.

Simpson, W.S., & Ramberg, J.A. (1997). The influence of religion on sexuality:

Slowinski, J.W. (1997). Sexual adjustment and religious training: A sex therapist's perspective. In J.S. Hyde & J. DeLamater (Eds.)., *Understanding human sexuality (6th ed)*. (pp. 137-154). Dubuque, IA: McGraw Hill.

Implications for sex therapy. In J.S. Hyde & J. DeLamater (Eds.)., *Understanding human sexuality (6th ed)*. (pp. 155-165). Dubuque, IA: McGraw Hill.

Stevens, S.R., Caron, S.L., & Pratt, P. (2003). Decade in review: The importance of religion in shaping the sexual attitudes of college students in the 1990's.

Strauss. G.H. (2001). "The real thing": A perspective on sexual revolution and a challenge to Christian professionals. *Journal of Psychology and Theology, 30,* 144-157.

Tiefer, L., & Kaschak, E. (Eds.) (2001). *A new view of women's sexual problems.*
Binghamton, New York: Haworth Press.

Timmerman, J.H. (1992). *Sexuality and spiritual growth.* New York: Corssroad.

Townsend, L. K. (2001). Embodiment versus dualism: A theology of sexuality from a
holistic perspective. *Review and Expositor, 98,* 157-172

Wolf, N. (1997). *Promiscuities: The secret struggle for womanhood.* New York: Ran-
dom House.

Zeiger, R.B. (1995). Reflections on infertility. In K. Weiner & A. Moon (Eds.), *Jewish
women speak out: Expanding the boundaries of psychology* (pp. 77-98).

Index